EASY EMDR

FOR CHILDREN AND ADULTS

THE HOME ANXIETY TREATMENT

EMDR IS RECOMMENDED BY THE WORLD HEALTH ORGANISATION

(and many other national clinical bodies)

"Children are highly susceptible to EMDR, the complexity comes with engaging the child's mind with suitable play to be able to understand and adhere to the process".

Dr Francine Shapiro PHD founder of EMDR - New York Times

An estimated 128 million children and adults globally are suffering from mental health problems at home, school and work, with anxiety & associated symptoms and disorders such as Stress, Anxiety, Eating Disorders, Post Traumatic Stress and Post Traumatic Stress Disorder, Depression, Anger, Behavior Issues, Addictions, IBS, Bereavement & more. Help is now here!

EMDR is a recommended treatment for anxiety disorders and post-traumatic stress. Our global mental health change initiative makes EMDR affordable to the masses for home use, to reach 20 million children globally.

EASY EMDR FOR 'EVERYONE EVERYWHERE'

(Part of the EASY EMDR Series)

ADRIAN RADFORD-SHUTE DHP Acc. Hyp

www.EASYEMDR.org

Copyright © 2012 Adrian Radford-Shute DHP Acc. Hyp.

All rights reserved.

ISBN: 9781790742714

By use of this material you agree to do so at your own risk and to indemnify the Author against accident or injury caused as a direct or indirect result of the use of the treatments or therapies contained herewith and by its use. If in doubt always seek medical advice.

DEDICATION

To the children in my life Hazel, Annie, and Jack

CONTENTS

	Acknowledgments & How to Use this Book	Pg 7
	Foreword & Introduction	Pg 9
1	Why Children & Parents need Help	Pg 20
2	What is EMDR?	Pg 38
3	What are the risks associated with EMDR?	Pg 44
4	Simple EMDR for Single Trauma	Pg 46
5	How Anxiety develops from Multiple Trauma	Pg 56
6	Understanding the basics of EMDR	Pg 76
7	The simple 4 step EMDR process	Pg 80
8	Step 1 – 'Find' for Adults	Pg 86
9	Step 1 – 'Find' for Older Children	Pg 116
10	Step 1 – 'Find' for Younger Children	Pg 142
11	Step 2 – 'Feel'	Pg 154
12	Step 3 – 'Follow'	Pg 168
13	Step 4 – 'Forget'	Pg 182
14	After EMDR – What next?	Pg 196
15	Conduct a Session for Adults	Pg 200
16	Conduct a Session for Older Children	Pg 226
17	Conduct a Session for Younger Children	Pg 254
18	Ongoing Therapy – Mindfulness and MindMagic	Pg 262
19	Anxiety & Depression Self Diagnostic Tests	Pg 272
20	Seeking Further Help & FAQ's	Pg 280

ACKNOWLEDGMENTS

With sincere thanks to Nick Fielding, author, journalist, explorer, a trusted loyal friend and confidant. Thank you for the guidance, knowledge, help and assistance in the editing and publication of this series of books for which I remain entirely grateful.

With sincere thanks to the founder and creator of EMDR Dr Francine Shapiro PhD. who is fully acknowledged and sincerely thanked for her development of the initial 8 stage EMDR protocol.

EASY EMDR is the vital next step in the natural evolution of this breakthrough treatment to ensure access is now made available for Everyone Everywhere. Without her initial work this would not have been possible, for which I hope mankind for ever more will one day become eternally grateful, as I am, for EMDR saved my life.

How to Use This Book

EASY EMDR for children has been developed, written and rigorously tested to ensure you can effectively carry out the treatment of EMDR at home by simply following these instructions:

1. First READ the entire book cover to cover.
2. Return to the Relevant Sections for ADULT Treatment and PRACTICE on an ADULT in SLOW TIME first.
3. Once you feel competent, return to the relevant sections for children and practice on an ADULT as if they were a child.
4. Once you feel competent begin treating Children and/or Adults.
5. Use the short condensed guides or 'TREATMENT SCRIPTS' at the back of the book, cross-referencing to any sections necessary.
6. Help and Guidance is covered in the FAQ section.
7. Pre and Post Treatment Tests are at the rear of the book.
8. For further help or support visit www.EASYEMDR.org.

For further reading please refer to the complete EASY EMDR series, with specific focused titles for Adult subjects or for clinical professionals wishing to learn or develop further knowledge.

CAUTION

If you or someone you know is in crisis or thinking of suicide seek professional help urgently – do not rely solely on this book:

Call your Doctor - or

Call the Emergency Services for your country - or

Go to the nearest Emergency Room - or

If services do not exist seek assistance from a responsible adult

Foreword

EMDR for EVERYONE EVERYWHERE (Eye Movement Desensitisation and Reprocessing) is the long-awaited home-based treatment for mental health issues by everyday people. It is one of a series of nine, released to finally resolve the age old problem of emotional trauma & anxiety with a 21st century clinical solution!

EASY EMDR for CHILDREN and PARENTS is for adults to use to treat children and adults with the clinically evidenced treatment referred to as **Eye Movement Desensitisation and Reprocessing** (EMDR), a ground breaking and rapidly growing treatment for generalised anxiety, emotional trauma, anger, panic attacks, bereavement, addiction (to alcohol, drugs, gambling, etc.) IBS, and many other similar conditions. EMDR is reported to also be helpful in managing the daily anxiety and anger related to Autism, Asperger, ADD, ADHD and Trauma in children.

EMDR is recommended by the World Health Organisation, The American Psychiatric Association, The UK National Institute for Health and Care Excellence, and many other global health institutions for the treatment of Post-Traumatic Stress Disorder (PTSD) and associated anxiety disorders.

The **EASY EMDR for EVERYONE EVERYWHERE** series provides solutions that can help to resolve most of these physical and mental health issues. There are nine books in the series for adults & children.

EMDR was first developed in 1990 by Francine Shapiro Ph.D. as a form of psychotherapy, this treatment reprocesses raw memories found 'locked in' the brain, thus relieving the symptoms of post-traumatic stress. By relieving certain stresses, namely anxiety and depression, other negative or avoidance behaviours or addictions can be changed.

This book simplifies and explains EMDR in plain language using just FOUR simple and easy to learn steps.

EASY EMDR is primarily for parents and adults to use at home or in the community to treat adults and children, using 'Eye Movement Desensitisation and Reprocessing' (EMDR) It's quick, easy, simple to learn and practice, and we are going to show you how right here.

EASY EMDR can also be used by anyone else who needs to know how to carry out First Aid for the Mind, whether they are guardians, therapists, clinicians, teachers, care workers, community-based workers, NGO's, overseas doctors, armed forces & emergency service personnel or just family or friends.

MINDMAGIC™ is a unique specific add-on Memory Mapping and MINDFULNESS therapy within EASY EMDR for children. It's so simple it can be used by anyone, anywhere, at any time. But MINDMAGIC™ isn't just for kids! With these simple easy-to-follow, step-by-step instructions and practical demonstrations adults can also be treated, safely and effectively.

We are aware that EMDR now has far wider and even greater effects in the treatment of anxiety, associated disorders, behaviours and addictions as reported widely in global medical research studies.

With over 11 million children and 50 million adults in the UK alone, 24% of girls and 10% of boys will suffer from mental health issues by the age of 14 that could be treated by EMDR. That's over 3 million children that can be helped in the UK at home!

With 1 in 4 adults suffering from mental health problems, more than 12 million adults in the UK can also be helped with fast effective EMDR treatment. In America it's 1 in 5. Globally the number rises higher still.

We believe with EASY EMDR we can help the millions of people in the UK suffering from anxiety, potentially saving the NHS £3.7 billion.

At present EMDR is not available via the NHS. A private course of treatment (6-12 sessions' NICE guidelines) can cost over £1000, which means that the cost barrier to treatment prevents millions of people in the UK alone from dealing with their depression, anxiety and other mental health issues.

Knowledge of EMDR is not widespread. Even some GP's have never heard of it. Along time ago in history only those with a license from the Royal College of Physicians could practice medicine, They had all the knowledge, written in thick books in Latin that every day folk could not understand, rather like the few books available today on EMDR! Vital life improving and even life-saving knowledge of EMDR is out of reach to the everyday person, which is why most people outside of private medicine have never even heard of it. Let's change that now!

Adrian Radford-Shute DHP Acc. Hyp. the author of the EASY EMDR series and the founder of the MINDMAGIC and MINDFIT therapies, is a Specialist EMDR Therapist working with children, adults and military, police, fire and ambulance personnel. Adrian is an Armed Forces Veteran who has worked with police, government, military and intelligence services in the UK & US.

As a former EMDR patient Adrian is a survivor of complex PTSD trauma and non-family child abuse and owes his life to the treatment of EMDR by Edward SIM, a renowned EMDR therapist. Edward studied under Dr Francine Shapiro, the founder of the original 8-stage EMDR Protocol.

After successful treatment Adrian was inspired to help others and went on to study Clinical Hypnotherapy and then specialised in EMDR where Adrian now practices privately, whilst also working pro bon for schools and a children's charity. Adrian founded the UK's first and only FREE EMDR charity 'PTSD FREE'.

After four years of research and development Adrian has devised a simple playful way of engaging children (and adults) with EMDR called MINDMAGIC™ which actually uses wands, spells and real magic from the worlds of wizard's to engage the child's mind fully, the revolution called for by world leading experts in this field, and the evolution to break EMDR free from private medicine.

We, yes that's you and me (Adrian), are the first people in the world in the field of Mental Health to take the controlling power from physicians to share it with the everyday person, where it is needed most! But we are not the first to do this.

Nicolas Culpeper was in fact the first person to revolutionise medicine worldwide, sharing the power that comes from medical knowledge to all.

Culpeper's *The Complete Herbal – An English Physician* was published over 300 years ago. By writing it in simple English he became the first to take the power from the physicians and gave it back to what he called 'the common people'. He told them where to find medicinal plants and how to prepare their own medicine. Physicians were outraged but it was too late. Next to the Bible *The Complete Herbal* is the world's most widely printed book.

For the first time the people, instead of relying on physicians, could practice their own cures. And now so can you in the field of mental health by learning how to practice EASY EMDR for yourselves and others. This revolutionary EASY EMDR series is history repeating itself once again.

EASY EMDR is the long awaited revolution and evolution in the treatment of mental health issues that stem from Post-Traumatic Stress – a term often we associate with war veterans, but actually it's an illness that can affect us all. Simply put; if we experience an event in life that is traumatic, and after that event we are still experiencing bad or painful thoughts or memories then this is post event trauma – it remains 'traumatic' even after the event has ended.

If these memories keep disturbing us and continue to cause us 'stress' then this is 'post-traumatic stress' – without the D. If we look at what Post Traumatic Stress 'Disorder' is – with the D, simply put that's defined by the rapid onset of stress relating to a single intense incident of trauma. That's why we see so many war veterans or survivors of terrorist incidents with PTSD and emotional disorders.

But anyone in day-to-day general life can suffer from just Post-Traumatic Stress, which is simply defined as the accumulation of stressful experiences or events in life that all mount up, effectively leaving us with the same symptoms as if we had been diagnosed with PTSD itself. The diagnosis doesn't matter, as the treatment is the same regardless – and so too often are the symptoms.

Anyone suffering with post-traumatic stress for long enough will experience anxiety, that feeling of dread in our stomachs, our chest, our throats, our heads, that can prevent us as children or teenagers or adults from living healthy productive lives, free from fear and worry. Anxiety can lead to compulsive behaviors, addictions, unsafe choices, self-harm and thoughts of, or even actual suicide.

If left untreated it can sadly be a killer.

With little access and massive underfunding of mental health services in the western world, let alone developing and poverty-stricken countries, humankind is facing one of its biggest social challenges ever. That's the Problem, EASY EMDR is a solution!

This book the first of its kind to demystify all the confusing medical jargon. It is simple, clinically tested, easy-to-follow, easy-to-practice at home or in the community, by parents, guardians or clinicians for children and adults. This simple book is illustrated with easy-to-follow guides in how to carry out EMDR treatment effectively

This book will help you to recognise if a child has any of these issues. It can also be used a diagnostic tool with medically approved tests, and this book will then teach you how to effectively deal with them. It may help you prevent traumatic life events that happen in childhood being allowed to grow and manifest into much bigger problems as teenagers grow up into adulthood.

This is a must-have guide for everyone who wants to help relieve the symptoms of stress, anxiety and emotional and post-traumatic stress.

Due to the Amazon printing process it is not possible to print just the few needed pages in colour as this prints the whole book in colour even if the pages are just black and white, the cost of the book would then triple placing it out of the reach of most people, so in order to ensure access to the book is at an affordable level the book and these images are printed in black & white.

You can access the colour images for FREE on KINDLE (free with every paperback purchase) or at www.EASYEMDR.org where there are free colour images and online tutorials available to support this book making listening and learning even easier with simple-to-follow instructions.

Introduction

The comprehensive international picture of the mental health of children or adolescents aged 5 to 17 years shows a growing prevalence of mental health problems, with an ever-increasing impact of those problems on families, parents, carers and young people themselves and the role of health and education services in providing assistance. Here are some helpful facts:

Approximately one in seven children and young people have experienced a mental disorder in the past year. This is consistent across many international studies.

220,000 people in the UK alone are unable to leave their homes due to anxiety costing the UK NHS by 2020 an estimated £3.7 billon.

There is now a special focus on improving both prevention and treatment efforts for young people, with Mental Health Initiatives around the world. The need for refocused effort by governments and the broader community to develop systems to both prevent mental health problems and to respond early to problems when they emerge is paramount.

The rates for depression, self-harm and thoughts about suicide in teenagers are particularly worrying, with approximately one in ten indicating that they have engaged in self-harming behavior. Three quarters did so in the previous 12 months.

For teenage girls aged 16-17 years, nearly one in five were found to meet the clinical criteria for depression. Around one quarter of teenage girls in the 16-17 year age range reported deliberately injuring themselves at some point in their lives.

The rates for depression in 11-17 year old's were found to be higher when young people provided information themselves rather than when their parents and carers did so.

One third of 11-17 year-olds report they have been bullied, and those who went on to develop behaviour disorders further reported they were then bullied more often. Young people with major depressive disorders were roughly twice as likely to then bully someone else. And so the negative cycle goes on.

Low weight problem eating behaviors were reported by only 1% of 11-17 year-olds. Binge eating and purging were reported by 1.3% of 11-17 year-olds.

Smoking, alcohol and drugs have been used by a growing number of 13-17 year-olds. Smoking was higher for young people with major depressive disorder. Alcohol consumption was higher among young people with major depressive disorder. Drug use was far higher for young people with a major depressive disorder. Online gambling is now however the largest growing addiction faced by teenagers.

Internet use and or electronic gaming are also highly problematic for 11-17 year old's, affecting their ability to eat, sleep, and spend time with family, friends and doing homework.

Social Media is effecting nearly every child who is using it in many positive yet many negative ways as widely reported in the news.

This is an important signal to all parents who are faced with the challenging task of helping children navigate the transition from childhood to adulthood.

The very good news is that EMDR is a highly effective treatment and parents who want to take more responsibility for their children because they have perhaps been let down by local mental health services now can in the safety of their own home.

By making EMDR available for home use we have responsibly taken away the reliance on physicians and demystified the treatment right here for you, to learn in very simple quick easy steps, giving the power back to the everyday people, to help change how people around the world treat mental health at home and in their communities.

It doesn't necessarily remove the need or role of therapists in the treatment of complex anxiety and complex associated disorders, but for those who cannot afford such help or have little or no access to EMDR, this simple book can change and even save lives all around the world, and in developing countries where there is no access to EMDR or even therapists.

Even in developed countries at present it is a chance encounter or a post code lottery whether you will be able to access EMDR.

This book will now teach you:

- How to use EMDR (Eye Movement Desensitisation and Reprocessing) safely at home or in a non-clinical setting in a simplified and easy format.

- How to use simple psychotherapy techniques to unlock memories and trauma in children and adults safely without the need for medical training.

- How to use after these treatments, MINDFULNESS in a new simple way using 'Magical Spells' or MIND MAGIC to protect the mind from stress and trauma as life carries on positively.

This book is the first of its kind to bring together all these skill sets in simple to follow plain language. To make it even simpler there are further practical demonstrations available to accompany this book available at www.EASYEMDR.org.

Accessing the FREE online tutorials is not a requirement to learn EASY EMDR, it's just an added feature for those who'd like to learn more. This book has everything you will need to succeed even if you don't have internet access.

So here for the first time is the simple four step process:

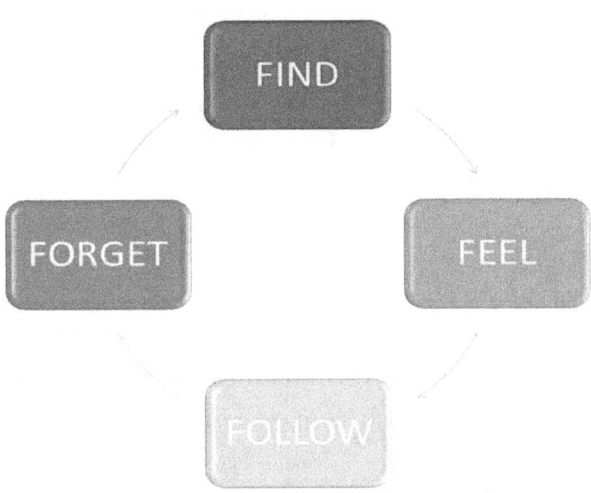

With this book you will also learn how to explain the concept of anxiety and stress to adults in plain language and children though magic and by using these magical spells how we can protect children's mind.

Don't be afraid about using these simple explanations, as educating older children about anxiety will teach them when to ask for help, before they self-harm or before their behaviours change. This education is vital in the early intervention of mental health and if you can teach your child how to recognise and ask for help early then you will be breaking the cycle of child and even adult mental health!

In this book you will find an easy simplified version of the EMDR clinical protocols that has been extensively clinically tested over 4 years of study on over 1000 adults and children in actual real time treatment, evidenced as being 99% effective by 1MIND.org in the resolution of post-traumatic stress and associated anxiety disorders and addictions.

In addition, you will also learn how to safely and effectively perform MEMORY MAPPING and MIND MAGIC, a 'history taking' therapy, extensively clinically tested, evidenced to be incredibly effective in the clinical treatment of over the 1000 adults and children, reported as being 100% effective in the non-verbal MAPPING of MEMORIES, which is detailed here again in a simple easy to follow step by step guide. It works every time on everyone!

Memory Mapping has been evidenced to reduce treatment time by up to 80%, because we are simply able to identify and then work on far more areas of trauma in a single session than any other protocol, to the extent a competent therapist can identify, target and resolve up to 10-15 separate memories of trauma per hour.

Over the four years of research conducted between 2014-2018, the greatest number of traumatic memories identified in a single session using this mapping method, was 72, with 28 of those traumatic memories being targeted and resolved fully with EMDR in a further single 1 hour session. Over 90% of all cases were resolved within 3-4 sessions. The clinical benefits of Memory Mapping is astounding.

Chapter 1

WHY CHILDREN & PARENTS NEED HELP

This book will explain in simple language why we may even need help. For an everyday person everything you may need to know I have endeavored to include here.

So to begin if we experience as we grow up from childhood unhealthy stress and anxiety, which is unresolved, we will take these experiences with us into adolescence and adult hood, where serious mental health issues may then develop and last for a life time. If these unhealthy beginnings can be identified and tackled early enough this negative cycle can be broken, which has been very hard if not impossible to do, until now with advent of EMDR.

In understanding where these problems stem from, right from the very start of life after we are born from 6 months to 2 years we naturally begin to experience stress and anxiety as we learn to become independent from our parents. We develop from being a baby into a child, conscious of our own ability to think and act independently. But after 2 years old we can become susceptible to external influences that prevent us from learning that it's ok to be separate from our family.

Perhaps our parents remain overly engaged in our lives, being too protective not allowing us to grow and develop as individuals, or perhaps our first experiences of growing up are the opposite, where neglect in its many forms may be experienced.

For a child growing up where there are no healthy boundaries anxiety can start to develop which can then be taken into adolescence and adult hood where very serious issues can then develop. These issues are referred to as varying Mental Health conditions or disorders.

Even for children growing up in a stable healthy balanced environment other external unwanted e.g. bereavement or emotional influences outside of the family unit can affect how a child develops and again anxiety can be learnt from a very young age.

As children grow into adolescence they can be susceptible to external unresolved influences of trauma, bereavement, abuse, neglect, bullying, sexuality confusion, social media or pressure to succeed and can begin to adopt unhealthy behaviors that are a cause for concern.

We can then take unresolved traumas from childhood into adulthood where they can manifest into chronic anxiety, depression, social phobias, varying disorders and emotional and psychological issues. Sometimes in adult hood we can also experience traumas so severe that we manifest the same symptoms and behaviors even without experiencing childhood trauma. The results can be the exact same.

Either way it's a problem that is vastly increasing and so EASY EMDR and MINDMAGIC have been developed and released as therapies to help where possible stop this in its tracks, whether in childhood, adolescence or later on in adulthood.

EMDR has been evidenced by the National Institute for Mental Health as being far superior to drug therapy, in a recent study that compared 8 sessions of EMDR treatment to 8 weeks of Fluoxetine (anti-anxiety) drug therapy, at the end of the trial – 91% of the

EMDR group reported no symptoms of PTSD, whereas only 74% reported changes in the Fluoxetine group. There were no side effects reported in the EMDR group, whereas the Fluoxetine group suffered headaches, dizziness, nausea and stomach upset for 8 weeks!

The original 8 phase EMDR protocol is considered highly complex, so much so even clinicians and therapists have been reluctant to study. In some countries you need a PHD in order to study EMDR. As such EASY EMDR and MINDMAGIC™ can help resolve this.

The formal clinical guidelines for EMDR therapist's state 6-12 sessions of EMDR may be required per client, and there is now a move to even increase this to 18 sessions putting the treatment even further out of the reach of the everyday child, adult and family.

It's one of the main reasons people face, who need help when seeking EMDR treatment – it's simply unaffordable to most.

With EASY EMDR and the process I use daily in my private clinics I rarely see patients for more than two to four 1 hour sessions – some I even see only once! Why? Because the system contained here, which uses the same 8 stage recommended original EMDR protocol as a base, is safely speeded up. Irrelevant material is cut out, and the initial phases that identify the trauma, or what is going to be worked on, are identified using a specialist far quicker therapy instead.

MEMORY MAPPING is a therapy that vastly speeds up the identification of conscious and even subconscious memories, thoughts or feelings within minutes. It is evolved from the base protocols of mindfulness another recommended therapy for anxiety.

MEMORY MAPPING is one of a number of aspects that makes this book unique, it will revolutionise ability to practice EMDR at home.

And to solve the original question posed by Dr. Francine Shapiro concerning the complexity that comes with engaging the child's mind with suitable play to be able to understand and adhere to the process, we have devised and clinically tested a new children's version of Memory Mapping and EMDR using wands, spells and magic from the world of wizard's. *"Using the wands and spells as you do is simply genius"* writes one parent.

The search for magical knowledge has obsessed humans since time gone by. The relationship between magic and science particularly in the early modern period is extremely important, as we asked what powers are out there that we can harness and adapt for our own use, and to some extent that is a form of magic.

Children believe in magic because they are starting to make sense of and control their world around them and they see it in films and TV!

We can use this belief to instill immediate confidence and trust in the EMDR treatment through magical play which engages the child's mind, essential for the resolution of trauma and anxiety.

EASY EMDR using MINDMAGIC™ will teach you how. You can now become a real life Witch or Wizard and use these spells to heal your own children, family and friends. As your children grow up perhaps most importantly of all, you can impart these skills onto them so they too can grow up to master EASY EMDR using MINDMAGIC™ healing future generations of their and your family.

It has been widely reported internationally children and adolescents in low-income families, with parents and carers with lower levels of education and with higher levels of unemployment have higher rates of mental disorders in the previous 12 months, and higher rates of associated behavior disorders.

The health systems, education and welfare sectors are critical in responding to the needs of children and young people with mental health problems and still have a key role to play, but they remain overburdened and underfunded even in the most developed of countries, and even then EMDR is rarely available.

So prevention at home and early intervention to reduce the prevalence and impact of mental health problems in our young and adult populations can now be taken on by families at home because if families could help themselves with the right tools they would.

In order to understand how as non-medical personnel we can actually use these tools, the first thing to understand is that this is EASY! There is no need to be fearful, EASY EMDR is SO simple families are using these skills right now to treat anxiety disorders with no medical knowledge other than what they've learnt here.

So perhaps it is important to first understand what are the most common disorders and the impact they can have on children, adolescents and adults.

Simply put Anxiety Disorders cause anxiety. They can be related to social phobias, a fear of social situations and interacting with other people, which can be caused by a fear of being judged in all areas of a person's life.

Separation anxiety disorder causes anxiety where an individual negatively experiences separation from home or from people to whom the individual has a strong emotional attachment, like a mother or father or even a pet.

Generalised anxiety disorder caused by a build-up of stress and worry causes anxiety where the person feels constantly anxious in a high state of stress.

Obsessive-compulsive disorders (OCD's) cause anxiety where a person feels the need to check things repeatedly, perform certain rituals repeatedly or experience certain thoughts repeatedly, in order try and control the environment around them.

Major depressive disorder is better known as Depression, or chronic sadness characterised by at least two weeks of low mood that is present across most situations.

It is often accompanied by low self-esteem, loss of interest in normally enjoyable activities, low energy and in some cases even pain without a clear cause – or psychosomatic pain.

Attention-Deficit/Hyperactivity Disorder (ADHD) is characterised by having problems paying attention, excessive activity or difficulty controlling behavior which is not appropriate for a person's age.

Interestingly ADHD can often be mistaken for Post-Traumatic Stress Disorder, which is a disorder characterised by a single traumatic event rather than an accumulation of life events that cause post-traumatic stress without the addition of the disorder.

Where ADHD is thought to be present the alternative of PTSD should always be explored at the same time – have the symptoms come from trauma?

Conduct disorder is characterised by inappropriate conduct for the situation relating to age whether that be anger or rage or sexual behavior, undressing in public, and may be caused by trauma, abuse or early sexualisation.

Almost one in seven 4-17 year-olds were assessed as having mental disorders, the equivalent to 128 million children and adolescents globally. This is the true scope of what could be treated with EASY EMDR.

Studies have concluded males are more likely than females to have experienced mental health disorders. ADHD was the most common mental health disorder in children and adolescents, followed by anxiety disorders, major depressive disorders and conduct disorders.

Almost one third of children and adolescents with a disorder, in fact had two or more mental disorders at some time in the previous 12 months. Adolescents were almost three times more likely to experience a severe mental disorder.

Sadly one in sixteen (6.2%) 4-17 year-olds with mental disorders were admitted to hospital, or attended emergency or outpatient departments in the previous 12 months.

In some developed countries schools have been placed at the forefront of providing access to services to around 40% of children and adolescents with mental health disorders where such services exist as these are often also massively underfunded. These range from individual counselling, group counselling or support programs, using a special class or school, seeing a school nurse or accessing other school services – but only where they are available.

A wide range of services should be available to assist young people with emotional and behavioral problems including health, school, telephone counselling and online services used by young people. Sadly gaining access to these services may take months if they can be accessed at all. In some countries where this book can perhaps also make a difference, these services simply do not exist what so ever.

So to help bridge this gap for the first time ever with EASY EMDR you can now take responsibility and help the children and adults you care for, to lessen the burden on young people and the health and welfare services that are reported almost daily now as struggling to cope to meet demand – and even so they still do not use EMDR!.

It feels like every day on national and local news very sad stories are told by individuals, families and charities of the failings of mental health services, but there is never any mention of what can be done to help these people. EMDR therapists and doctors around the world share in the frustration that this highly effective clinical treatment has not been widely publicised, and that children and adults need not suffer any more, but only if they can access affordable EMDR.

Well here you can. With the evolution of EASY EMDR it has now become, affordable, simple and easy to learn how to use at home or in the community, the unique treatment of EMDR to reduce anxiety.

EASY EMDR bridges the gap between private professional treatment and home therapy – this could therefore be considered as First Aid Treatment for the Mind!

In fact it's SO simple as you will see, the actual EMDR Treatment itself is ONLY one step! The initial steps are not in fact EMDR, they are just the steps to identify what to work on to make the subject feel well again. The final step is to ensure the treatment has worked and what to do if it needs a little 'tweak' here and there - it really is THAT EASY! And the EMDR phase is just making sure the subject's left and right brain is stimulated, by eye movement, touch or sound, where the subject follows your fingers left to right, or by you clicking to the left and right of the head, or tapping their knees, when thinking about the memory identified in the first stages – that's it!

The traditional EMDR process uses an EIGHT step protocol, it's important to understand that this model hasn't been changed or altered, it's just been simplified and in doing so a few tips have been added in the guides that will make the process even easier to learn. For therapists, clinicians or medical professionals or those wishing to change career to practice EMDR, or just those interested to learn more, perhaps you'd like to read the original eight step protocol and how this compares to the simplified four step process above which I've detailed at the rear of the book. But do you need to know this as a parent, friend, or family member to practice simple EMDR – NO!

With a complete quick and easy to follow step by step break down of each sequence this guide also contains an alternative step by step guide for older children to bring to life the world of 'wizarding magic' in an exciting and easy to imagine process for children. For younger children there is also a separate guide on how to use finger puppets and play to help the little ones recover from anxiety and trauma.

Now you can go on to learn how to use wands and magical circles and crystal balls and finger puppetry to extract distressing thoughts from the mind and examine them externally.

When they are in this external form the fear of those distressing or 'excess' memories and the emotional attachment can be reduced.

Our minds are programmed to 'process' experiences of traumatic memories to ensure we learn from them and use the wisdom of experience to keep us safe in the future, so why does this often not work and why does counselling or talking therapy often not work?

Processing might take 1 minute, 1 hour, 1 day, 1 week or 1 month, but if it takes longer than 3 months – this is the magical time frame, the memory will become 'locked in' our mind. We now know after 25 years of mental health study that once trauma is 'locked in' it stays there forever, locked deep within the mind and no matter what we do that part of our mind becomes stuck at the age the trauma happened.

I explain it's like an Application or APP running in the background of a 'smartphone' that hasn't been turned off. If there are enough Apps running silent in the background they start to drain the phones battery, everything starts to slow down, the phone plays up doing weird unexplained things until eventually the phones battery gives up.

Our own minds operate just like smartphones. This is why therapy and counselling for trauma rarely works and isn't recommended for unresolved trauma **beyond 3 months**. Therapy and counselling helps us to process the immediate trauma but we now know we have to access those services within the magical window of 3 months, and we all know just how hard it can be outside of private medicine to get to see a counsellor or have any kind of therapy within 3 months if at all. It may take months using up the vital window of opportunity. This is why national clinical bodies such as NICE in the UK recommend EMDR for trauma beyond **3 months**.

But if a child's minds is still developing and therefore cannot understand what's happened or the memory is too painful, then it can become locked in at the age of the actual memory regardless of the 3 month point or not!

This also often depends on the adult's reaction around the time of the trauma. Often we see adults 'teach' their children anxiety.

Anxiety is a learned behaviour!

This is why it is so important when treating any child the parents also look inwardly at themselves and use this EMDR to treatment to resolve their own fears and anxiety lead behaviors where this is needed, to heal the family as a whole. This is a major contributor to the increase in global mental health cases. Healing the family as a whole is one of the most important aspects of this book hence the book name EASY EMDR for EVERYONE EVERYWHERE.

But in some communities, refugee camps or countries as a whole there simply aren't any councilor or therapists. In developing countries or those ravaged by war or natural disaster only basic health services may exist. Doctors may already be overburdened, but it is imaginable that other staff and community workers can now step in.

Einstein once said "Imagination is more powerful than knowledge".

Imagine the good that could come from these books being used to heal mental wounds of war and displacement experienced by children and adults in refugee camps and orphanages around the world?

We can, which is why for every 10 books bought we are donating the funds for 1 book to be printed free by UNICEF distribution centers and our partners to reach these areas. With grants we could do more.

Let's not forget in the developed world each year children experience violence and disaster and face other traumas even at home or at school. Young people are injured, they see others harmed by violence, they suffer sexual abuse, and they lose loved ones or witness other tragic and shocking events.

Parents and caregivers with EMDR can help children overcome these experiences or 'traumas' and start the process of recovery at any time.

Trauma is often thought of as physical injuries when you break a bone etc. Psychological trauma is the result of an emotionally painful, shocking, stressful, and sometimes life-threatening experience. It may or may not involve physical injuries, but can also result from witnessing distressing events.

I've treated many children who have seen such events only on TV or the News, but the affects have been the same, whether witnessed first-hand or through broadcast or social media which is rapidly growing in causation. Examples include natural disasters, building fires, reports of physical or sexual abuse, and terrorism – all things children perhaps shouldn't really see or bare witness to.

Watching disasters such as hurricanes, earthquakes, and floods which can claim many lives, destroy homes or whole communities, can cause serious psychological trauma in children, which can also be caused by acts of violence or seeing anger in the home around them.

The September 11, 2001 terrorist attack on the World Trade Centre in New York is but one example of many. Mass shootings in schools or communities and physical or sexual assault are other common examples. The Grenfell Tower fire in London is yet another where I have personal experience of treating 'TV witnesses' to those events.

Traumatic events can seriously threaten a child's and of course even an adults own sense of safety, or perhaps the child becomes overwhelmed in fear of losing their parents when they go to work to a terrorist incident, accident or disaster. The good news is children with such symptoms can recover fully and quickly with EMDR.

Reactions or responses to trauma can be immediate or delayed. Reactions to trauma differ in severity and cover a wide range of behaviors and responses. Children with existing mental health problems, past traumatic experiences, and/or limited family and social support may be more reactive to trauma.

Frequently I've seen and experienced responses from children after trauma with a loss of trust and a fear of the event happening again no matter how unlikely as adults we know that to be. It is much harder for a developing child's mind to process or make sense of the actuality reality of a situation. But it can much easier to heal a child mind when compared to an adults. Children's minds are like ink on blotting paper which can be wiped away quickly without leaving a stain as it hasn't had sufficient time to dry in to the paper, whereas with an adults mind the ink has had far more time to dry, and so it can take a little longer to resolve, but we are only talking hours here!

It's important with children to remember:

- Children's reactions to trauma are strongly influenced by an adults response
- People from different cultures have their own way of reacting to trauma
- Children react differently to trauma based on age and gender

Here are some commonly experienced responses to trauma among children:

Children age 5 and under may react in a number of ways including:

- Showing signs of fear
- Clinging to parent or caregiver
- Crying or screaming
- Whimpering or trembling
- Moving aimlessly
- Becoming immobile
- Returning to behaviours common to being younger
- Thumb sucking
- Bedwetting
- Being afraid of the dark

Children age 6 to 11 may react by:

- Isolating themselves
- Becoming quiet around friends, family, and teachers
- Having nightmares or other sleep problems
- Refusing to go to bed
- Becoming irritable or disruptive
- Having outbursts of anger or starting fights
- Being unable to concentrate
- Refusing to go to school
- Complaining of physical problems
- Developing unfounded fears
- Becoming depressed
- Expressing guilt over what happened
- Feeling numb emotionally
- Doing poorly with school and homework
- Losing interest in fun activities
- Thumb sucking and bed wetting

Adolescents age 12 to 17 may react by:

- Having flashbacks to the event (flashbacks are the mind reliving trauma)
- Having nightmares or other sleep problems
- Avoiding reminders of the event
- Using or abusing drugs, alcohol, or tobacco
- Being disruptive, disrespectful, or behaving destructively
- Having physical complaints
- Feeling isolated or confused
- Being depressed
- Being angry
- Losing interest in fun activities
- Having suicidal thoughts

Adolescents may feel guilty. They may feel guilt for not preventing an injury or someone's death.

Perhaps with this knowledge in hindsight the abuse I suffered as child by a non-family member could have been identified and stopped much sooner by my parents, but it wasn't as through no thought of their own no one ever taught them to look out for these indicators.

In fact it's only now that our generation has become open to speaking out about abuse and trauma, rather than "we don't talk about that" a learned behavior of many adults after the first and second World Wars, which is why now we are seeing such a massive increase in the counts of reported abuse and anxiety related disorders and mental health services are overburdened where funding hasn't caught up. The vast majority of these cases can be traced all the way back to the learned behaviours that once helped our parents and grandparents cope with the aftermath of war, it isn't their fault either!

So what can parents now do differently to help?

After violence or disaster, parents and family members should identify, express and address their own feelings to allow them to help others. Then explain to children what happened and let them know:

- You love them
- The event was not their fault
- You will do your best to take care of them
- It's okay for them to feel upset

Do:

- Allow children to cry
- Allow sadness to be expressed
- Allow anger to be expressed (but not played out in rage)
- Let children talk about feelings
- Let them write about feelings
- Let them draw pictures about the event or their feelings (we can use these later when we introduce THERAPLAY as part of EMDR)

Don't:

- Expect children to be brave or tough
- Make children discuss the event before they are ready
- Get angry if children show strong emotions
- Get upset if they bed wet, act up or thumb suck

If children have trouble sleeping give them extra attention, let them sleep with a light on, or let them sleep in your room (for a short time). You can also use the MINDMAGIC therapy which is MINDFULNESS for children found and fully explained at the end of this book.

Try to keep to normal routines, for example, reading bedtime stories, eating dinner together, watching TV together, reading books, exercising or playing games. If you can't keep to normal routines, make new ones together as a whole family.

Help children feel in control when possible by letting them choose meals, pick out clothes, or make some decisions for themselves.

Helping children with these simple basics can start immediately, even at the scene of the event. Most children recover within a few weeks of a traumatic experience, while some may need help longer. Grief, a deep emotional response to loss, may take months to resolve. Children may experience grief over the loss of a loved one, friend or even pets. Bereavement is very commonly experienced by children.

It's important to identify those children who need extra support and help them obtain it. Some children may need help from a mental health professional. Some people may seek other kinds of help from teachers or community leaders but how will you know this?

If the child is attending school perhaps speak to a teacher, often in schools we now find dedicated staff trained to help.

If you cannot find the support or there isn't access to any help, or the only help available is privately and you would find it hard to fund treatment, then this may be the book you've always been waiting for, it's certainly what it's been designed for!

If there's a long wait to see a mental health professional then there's certainly no harm in treating children at home as an early intervention with this simple four step EASY EMDR process so why wait, why prolong a child's pain?

It's important to monitor problematic behaviours which could be:

- Refusing to go to places that remind them of the event
- Emotional numbness or unexplained anger/rage
- Behaving dangerously
- Sleep problems including nightmares

Always pay even closer attention to children who have suffered trauma:

- Listen to them
- Accept/don't argue about their feelings
- Help them cope with the reality of their experiences

By doing simple things like these it can reduce or prevent memories of trauma being 'locked in' as we've discussed. You can at that time also help avoid memories becoming 'locked in' by reducing other stress a child may experience at the same time, which only serves to increase their anxiety such as;

- Frequent moving or changes in place of residence
- Long periods away from family and friends
- Pressures to perform well in school
- Nagging at home over basic ideals such as a tidy room
- Fighting within the family
- Being hungry

Parents and caregivers should also strictly limit or prevent viewing of repetitive news reports about traumatic events. Young children may not understand that news coverage is about one event and not multiple similar events and they might think it's where they live!

Above all else it's important if you want to avoid traumatic memories being locked in, if faced with immediate trauma:

Don't:

- Force people to tell their stories
- Probe for personal details
- Say things like "everything will be OK," or "at least you survived"
- Say what you think they should feel or have acted
- Say people suffered because they deserved it
- Be negative about available help
- Make promises that you can't keep such as "you'll go home"

Even if you do abide by all of these we know that some children may still have prolonged mental health problems after a traumatic event. These may include grief, depression, anxiety, and post-traumatic stress disorder (PTSD). Some trauma survivors get better without support. Others may need care or even prolonged help from a professional mental health strategy.

If after a month in a safe environment children are not able to perform normal routines or new behaviour or emotional problems develop, then contact a health professional and/or use EASY EMDR.

It's common for children and even adults to react the same if they are subjected to the exposure of the same traumatic event, adults too may often need the help that EASY EMDR can give them.

Always look out for your own wellbeing as well as that of any children especially when some of what I have listed here as occurred:

- Being directly involved in the trauma, especially as a victim
- Severe and/or prolonged exposure to the event
- Personal history of prior trauma
- Family or personal history of mental illness
- Severe behavioural problems
- Limited social support; lack of caring family and friends
- Ongoing life stressors such as moving to a new home or new school, divorce, job change, or financial troubles

Some symptoms may require immediate attention from a mental health professional especially if these symptoms involve:

- Flashbacks
- Racing heart and sweating
- Being emotionally numb
- Being extremely sad or depressed
- Feeling suicidal or expressing thoughts to end life

To determine if you need help with any of these symptoms there are easy to use clinical self-diagnostic tests (GAD-7 and PHQ-9) at the end of the book, and then seek medical help or advice as guided in the test outcomes and actions referred to. Remember if you have serious concerns or are in any doubt always seek urgent medical help.

With mental health services being critically underfunded, or simply just not affordable or available in some communities and countries, then EMDR is widely recognised by all clinical bodies as a suitable immediate intervention, but with access to such therapists either unaffordable, rare or completely non-existent, then this book may just be the long term, affordable and positive complete solution you and your family been looking for. After all according to the National Institute for Mental Health it is 91% effective, and in our clinical studies with this particular system it is recorded 99% effective.

You have nothing to lose but everything to gain by using EASY EMDR. So lets take a look at what exactly EMDR is and how it works.

Chapter 2

What is EMDR?

If something traumatic has happened to you, whether it be a car accident, abuse or something seemingly less significant like being humiliated, the memory of your experience may come crashing back into your mind, forcing you to relive the original event with the same intensity of feeling - like it's actually taking place in the present moment at that very time and for real.

These experiences that pop into your awareness may present themselves as either flashbacks or nightmares (they can often come at night) and are thought to occur because the mind was simply too overwhelmed during the event to process what was going on. If enough of these events throughout life are not processed, or the event itself is so traumatic, the mind can become overloaded leading to mental breakdown or self-harm as a defence mechanism.

As a result, these unprocessed memories and the accompanying sights, sounds, thoughts and feelings are stored in the brain in their 'raw' form, where they can be accessed each time we experience something that triggers a recollection of the original event.

While it isn't possible to fully erase these memories, the process of **Eye Movement Desensitisation & Reprocessing (EMDR)** can alter the way these traumatic memories are stored within the brain - making them easier to manage and causing you far less distress - if any at all.

EMDR is a form of psychotherapy developed in the 1980s by the American psychologist Dr. Francine Shapiro. During a stroll in the park, Francine said she made a chance observation that certain eye movements appeared to reduce the negative emotion associated with her own traumatic memories. When she experimented, she found that others also exhibited a similar response to eye movements, and so she set about conducting controlled studies before developing what she called 'a multiphase approach to trauma reduction'.

Today, the treatment is used to treat a wide range of psychological difficulties that typically originate in trauma, such as direct or indirect experiences of violence, accidents or natural disaster.

EMDR is also used to treat more prolonged, low-grade distress that originates in shock or loss and/or issues experienced during life.

The experiences outlined above often lead to a post-traumatic stress disorder diagnosis, for which EMDR has been recommended by the National Institute of Health and Care Excellence (NICE), The World Health Organisation & the American Psychiatric Association, and Government Defence and Veterans departments around the world.

Anyone suffering from Post-Traumatic Stress (you do not have to be diagnosed as having a Disorder) will benefit from EMDR treatment.

Increasingly, EMDR treatment is also being widely and successfully used and reported as the 'go to' treatment for many other anxiety related issues, because they are often caused by Post-Traumatic Stress.

These are widely reported in EMDR research and studies to include:

- Depression
- Suicidal Thoughts
- Self-Harm
- Anxiety – General & Social
- Phobias
- Fears
- Stress
- Anger
- Insomnia
- Panic Attacks
- Bereavement
- Addictions
- Obsessive Compulsive Disorders (OCD)
- Eating Disorders
- Irritable Bowel Syndrome (IBS)
- Fibromyalgia
- Chronic Pain Disorder (CPD)
- Low Self Esteem
- Lack of Confidence
- Body Dysmorphia

Of note I have had complete success treating ALL of these issues, symptoms, disorders and conditions with EMDR in a clinical setting. I have also had success in teaching the everyday person to do exactly the same in a non-clinical setting. The difference is... well there isn't one, that's why you can learn this too!

When traumatic events occur, the body's natural thought processing and coping mechanisms can be overwhelmed and subsequently the memory is inadequately processed and stored incorrectly.

The goal of EMDR treatment is to replicate REM (Rapid Eye Movement) sleep whilst awake, to properly process these traumatic memories, reducing their impact and helping clients to develop coping mechanisms.

This is done through a four-phase approach to address the past, present, and future aspects of a stored memory, requiring clients to recall distressing events safely while receiving bilateral sensory input – in other words rapid side to side eye movements (as if in REM Sleep), audible sounds or tapping.

The recalled memories are then Desensitised which allows new neurological pathways to form, effectively Reprocessing the emotional attachment to the event. All of which has been confirmed and evidenced by clinical and MRI study.

The goal of EMDR is simple - "to reduce distress in the shortest period of time using a comprehensive approach with therapeutic protocols and procedures".

There are traditionally eight phases to the EMDR therapy protocol but these can now be shortened safely to just 4 simple phases, reducing treatment time for children and adults.

EASY EMDR targets memories of trauma and it is these memories of trauma that when locked in can very often lead to anxiety and the associated disorders.

So once the memories have been treated with EASY EMDR and are no longer an issue for the subject, then what we see is an almost immediate and rapid decrease in the associated symptoms, disorders and even addictions.

The reported benefits of EMDR treatment are:

- Living free of Addictions and OCD's
- A reduction in re-experiencing traumatic memories
- Increase in energy and performance
- Feeling more able to cope with and manage traumatic memories without needing to avoid potential triggers
- Feeling more able to engage in and enjoy pleasurable activities and relationships

- Reduced feelings of stress, anxiety, irritation and hypervigilance
- Allowing you to rest well, address pressure and/or conflict
- Allowing you to go about your daily life without feeling fearful and prone to panic
- Reduced feelings of isolation, hopelessness and depression
- The ability to leave the home on your own without fear or anxiety
- A boost in self-confidence and self-esteem
- The ability to return to work with confidence and excitement
- A feeling of no longer being bothered about the past
- Effectively forgetting about previous traumatic events rather than the treatment erasing them -the effects however are the same
- A reduction or cessation in medication with the support of medical practitioners
- Improved relationships with children, siblings, adults, parents, partners, friends work colleagues and acquaintances

For some people just feeling lighter and no longer living with the guilt or shame of trauma or abuse is enough. Weight management becomes much easier, as does sleeping and as such the positive cycle of the benefits of EMDR can be felt to increase.

EMDR is not a 'panacea' or a fix for all solution for all mental health problems. EMDR is through research becoming far more widely understood and practiced and as such the number of emotional and physical problems it can be used for continues to grow.

We are also seeing a growing number of associated conditions where EMDR can help people manage living with chronic conditions such as HIV and Parkinson's attain a better quality of life, as EMDR can help people reduce the catastrophisation associated with a diagnosis.

EMDR can easily be used to eradicate fears and phobias in minutes, you just need to find the initial memory and target that! We call these single traumas and we're going to have a look at how to do that now.

Chapter 3

What are the risks associated with EMDR?

NONE

There are NO reported side effects or risks associated with EMDR, so even if you don't get it absolutely right first time or ever, you don't need to be perfect as you can't do any damage or harm with the home use of EMDR – so what do you have to lose? This is exactly why EASY EMDR is a breakthrough treatment and solution.

Chapter 4

Simple EASY EMDR - for Single Trauma

So now we know EMDR is the treatment for trauma, we can start by dividing trauma into two distinct categories: **Single & Multiple.**

So what's the difference? Single Trauma is just one episode, event, memory, fear or phobia. In contrast to treating Multiple Trauma this is really super quick and so easy to resolve.

I'm going to explain this here using the simple 4 step EASY EMDR process so you can try this on an adult straight away. This way you'll have a very basic understanding of what EMDR actually is and why it's really so simple.

Once you've experienced treating someone with EASY EMDR or perhaps you're the one whose been treated you will 100% <u>**know**</u> it works - because rather than taking my word for it you would have seen the actual process before, during and after and you'll be able to carry this new found understanding, knowledge and belief even further, to then be able and confident to go on and treat Multiple Trauma. So what is Multiple Trauma?

Multiple Trauma is a group of single traumas all stacked up on top of each other that are seemingly unconnected, but the more multiple traumas we 'lock in' the more we tend to attract! Single Trauma usually only manifests or ends up with a phobia e.g. fear of heights, spiders, dogs etc.

Multiple Trauma however can lead to generalised stress and anxiety, associated disorders or even addictions. So treating Multiple Trauma is approached in a little bit more depth for you here to cover most eventualities and outcomes. In order to still make treating Multiple Trauma simple and easy there's a bit more detail that will help in the chapters that follow. For now just to get you started, I'm going to explain in those 4 easy steps how to remedy single traumas, fears or phobias.

As Single Trauma is quite simple, as it relates to one single event, all your subject (that's going to be treated) needs to find is the MEMORY of that event or where it started. If they can do this easily then this very quick remedy below is suitable and perhaps all you will ever need. If not, do still read on without jumping to the Multiple Trauma chapter as knowledge of the basics here will help regardless.

To remind ourselves the basic 4 step process we're going to use is:

STEP ONE – FIND

Ask the subject to close their eyes and go to the memory of the event (in this illustration it's a memory of a fire). Ask them to tell you when they are there!

STEP TWO – FEEL

Ask the subject "where can you now feel that in your body?" They will point or say an area e.g. chest, tummy, head etc. That feeling is 'anxiety'! Now ask them to 'grade' that feeling on a scale of 0-10; 0 being low, 10 being high.

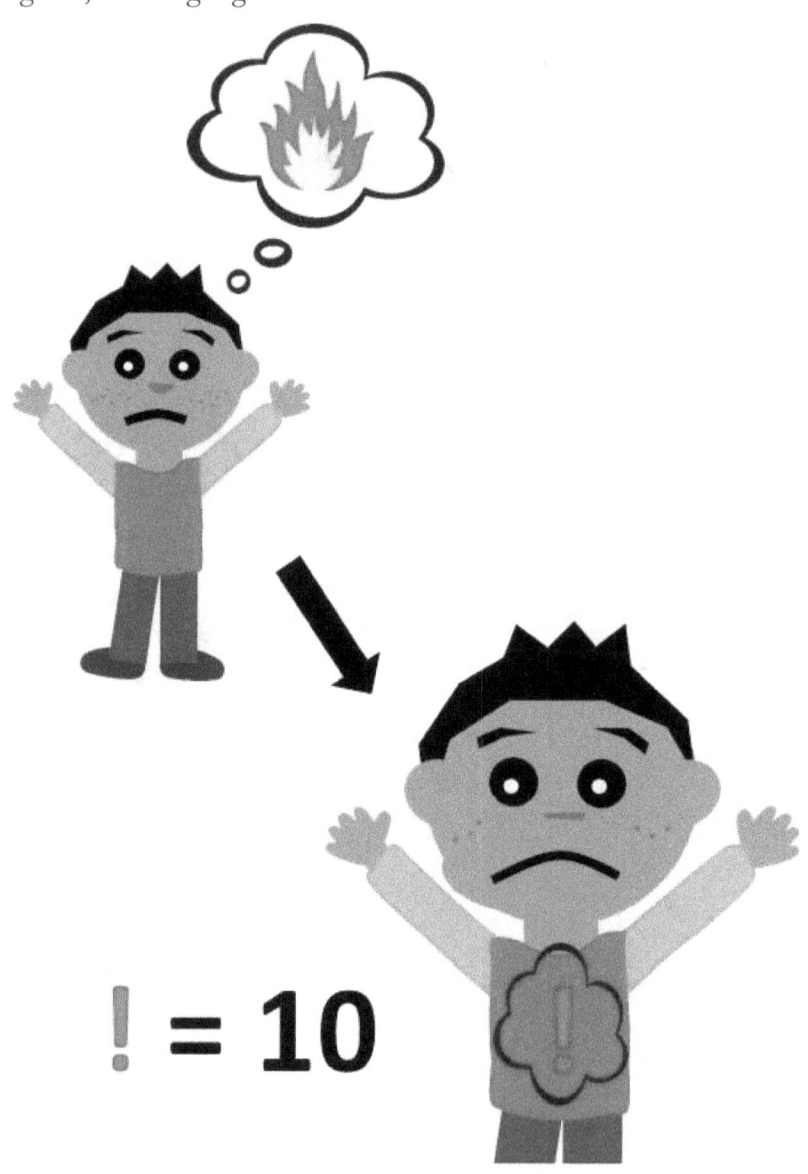

STEP THREE – FOLLOW

Once they have graded their feeling ask the subject to open their eyes and 'follow' your fingers with their eyes, remind them to still think of the memory, as you move your fingers them from left and right their eyes should track them, remind them to not move their head – just the eyes.

As the subject follows your fingers tell them the feeling (measured by the number) will now start to come down as they forget the emotion attached to it. Keep moving your fingers and keep asking "what has it come down to now" they should say a number lower than the first number they started at. Keep moving your fingers, keep checking in "what number has the old feeling gone down to" until the feeling reduces down again & again to zero!

STEP FOUR – FORGET

Ask the subject to now try and think of the OLD memory again and the OLD feeling, this time the memory may be there but the bad feeling has gone! Often the subject now feels positively different, sometimes even happy about the memory, that's when you will know the trauma has been forgotten.

If when the subject goes back into the memory and the feeling hasn't completely gone then just re-start the process again and keep going until it has completely gone. It's very common for this to happen and for the process to be repeated two, three or four times - so don't worry. When the subject goes back to the memory again re-check what number they grade the feeling at, it should be lower than the first number, keep moving your fingers from side to side ensuring the subject is keeping their head still and keep asking what the number has gone down to now. Again just keep going until it's finally resolved.

After you've carried out this basic EASY EMDR you can now do something highly positive with your subject to reinforce the effectiveness of the EMDR. Once your subject has forgotten or can't feel the 'old feeling', ask them to just go back and have a quick check - get them to close their eyes again and 'go back to the OLD memory'.

Now ask them "how good do you now feel on a different scale of 1-7"? If the answer is a 5, 6 or 7 then the trauma of that single memory is now resolved sufficiently.

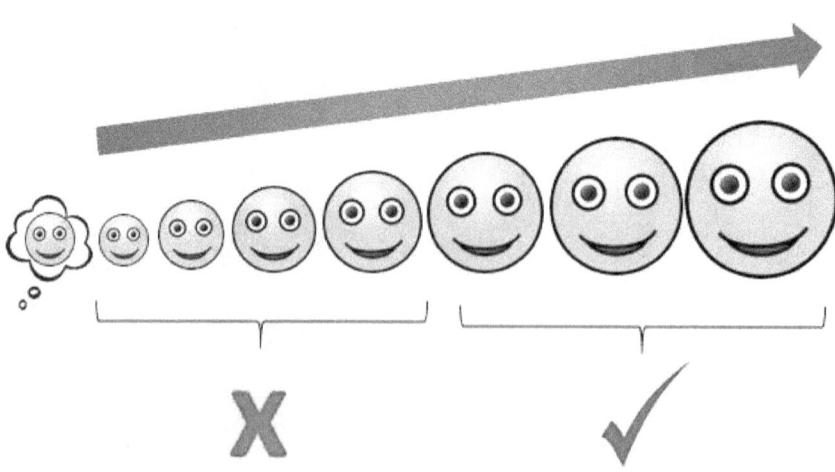

If the number they say is lower, in-between 1-4 don't worry, just read on as there is lots more information to help identify why that may be and how to treat that memory further.

Usually at this stage you are probably going to hear or see the excitement in your subject or yourself. This can be so very rewarding when you realise for the first time perhaps in your life or theirs, just how simple it is to resolve traumatic thoughts or reoccurring memories by moving your fingers and that you've made it happen!

It's at this point when that eureka moment happens, people start to realise just how easy EMDR can be and perhaps just how easy it is to build this into the daily schedule of life where needed, as easy as putting on a plaster! EASY EMDR for Single Trauma can be seen as 'first aid for the mind'! If you find traumas early enough and treat them as an early or emergency intervention, as mental health first aid, then they often never get worse or even return.

It's very common for Single Trauma to be resolved in this simple easy way. It doesn't take extensive training, expensive equipment, a complex academic understanding of psychology or medicine, or a clinical degree. Just follow the 4 easy steps FIND FEEL FOLLOW FORGET and say goodbye to trauma!

But what if you've gone through the above very simplified process and there hasn't been the resolution you'd expected. Perhaps when they go back to the memory to test if they can feel it they still can? This can also be common, and therefore perhaps a little more help is needed or perhaps there are in fact Multiple Traumas present that are preventing the resolution of a memory. If that's the case then just read on to see how to easily treat Multiple Trauma.

Chapter 5

How Anxiety develops from Multiple Trauma

So we have already learnt our minds are programmed to 'process' experiences of traumatic memories to ensure we learn from them and use the wisdom of experience to keep us safe in the future. To reiterate, processing might take 1 minute, 1 hour, 1 day, 1 week, 1 month, but if it takes longer than 3 months – this is the magical time frame, the memory will become 'locked in' deep within the mind, no matter what we do it will always be there unless we have been treated for Single Trauma as we've just covered. But if we haven't we can then develop generalised anxiety if all these anxieties group together, and it is often the accumulative effect that can cause much greater anxiety and associated disorders, distractive behaviours or addictions. This is what we call MULTIPLE TRAUMA.

I explain this in an easy way to my clients that it's like an Application running in the background of a 'smartphone' that hasn't been turned off. If there are enough Apps running in the background the battery starts to drain, everything starts to slow down and the phone starts to play up until eventually the phones memory shuts down. Our own minds are just like smartphones. And this is why therapy and counselling for trauma rarely works and isn't recommended for unresolved trauma **beyond 3 months** (UK NICE guidelines 2018).

Therapy and Counselling helps us to process the immediate trauma but we now know we have to access those services within the magical window of 3 months, and we all know just how hard it can be outside of private medicine to get to see a counsellor or have any kind of therapy. This is why national clinical bodies such as NICE in the UK recommend EMDR for trauma beyond **3 months**.

But if as a child our minds are still developing and we cannot understand what's happened or the memory is too painful then it can become locked in at that age of the actual memory regardless of the 3 month point or not! Again it's important to reiterate this often depends on the adult's reaction around the time of the trauma.

What I'm going to explain now is what I call the ANXIETY GRAPH, which will help explain this in more detail. It is an important part not to miss.

It's quite an in-depth explanation but again I've kept it simple to understand, but it's important to read as this forms the general understanding and explanation we can read out loud to any adult we are trying to help. It may also be suitable for adolescents if they are able to comprehend and are ultimately interested in learning about anxiety.

It isn't necessary to explain this to younger children and it won't affect the outcome of the treatment either way, but it can be very helpful for people to finally understand why they have been acting and feeling the way they do. It can be a massive sense of relief in my experience for most people.

It will explain a very simple analogy of how Anxiety develops, how it affects us, how we develop addictions or distraction behaviours, why and how prescription medications do and don't work and ultimately and why EMDR should be used as a treatment FIRST and why any therapy should be used AFTER and not before. This is one of the most powerful and empowering explanations I give to my clients.

Once they see this graph and how it really works in real life they always 100% guaranteed have that eureka moment!

It's like a light bulb goes on their head and finally they then get it too! They will then understand perhaps why months or even years with some cases of counselling why therapy has never worked for them and could never work for them. Clients always say to me 'why haven't I seen this before, why has this never been explained before and why doesn't everyone know about this!' It is recognised medically and referred to as Subject Units of Distress (SUDs) yet it only appears to be explained in private mental hospitals, until now.

It also helps us understand where other therapies such as Mindfulness fit in and why these should be used after EMDR as they are a 'coping mechanism' that needs to be practised every day to cope better with life's events. Some therapies are NOT treatments.

Even Cognitive Behavioural Therapy (CBT) takes much longer than EMDR and although it is also recommended by governing clinical bodies it is widely reported in many studies as non-effective as a long term solution – but why? Simple; because CBT doesn't resolve the 'locked in' memories of trauma.

CBT helps us look at them from a different perspective, but that takes much study, lots of evening homework and a calm mind, so when in the heat of experiencing anxiety, it takes much intellectual ability to learn, recall and apply the training and the focus to intervene. So what do the rest of us do?

Until now nothing! We were left with no other choice other than drug therapy and all the associated side effects. We've already discussed why the National Institute for Mental Health (NIMH) advocate EMDR as being far superior to even drug therapy, because EMDR targets the causes, it doesn't mask them! And here in this Anxiety Graph as it builds we can see how.

You should try drawing this yourself on a piece of A4 as we go along.

So on this graph we are going to start by drawing the axis, the lines; one up and down on the left and one along the bottom. Now we need to write along the bottom 25, 50, 75 and 100. That's how we're going to measure the level of anxiety.

And now on this graph we're going to put those 'Subjective Units of Distress' – SUD's; the building blocks of stress and anxiety.

When I'm in a session I always draw this graph upside down as its facing the client not me, you can try this too, it's very easy and I always have a little ice breaker with my clients that "as you can see I passed the upside down writing course... I got a B *not* an A!" – We don't have to be perfect! Do remember that as you learn to draw it.

We can explain as we go, that "now on this graph we're going to draw the first few building blocks". Draw them as rectangles on the graph base line between 0 and 25 one on top of the other. You can see them here in blue.

Make up an example that "perhaps somethings happened to us a child and we've a few bad experiences of something" these are trauma, represented here on the graph. Now it's useful to know and explain that 'trauma' is 'subjective', in other words a memory of something that is bad for one person might not be bad for someone else. Here you can give any simple non harmful example for instance; let's say I climbed a Cherry Tree when I was younger and it scared me and now I don't like cherries! We can put that on the graph as it scares me, it causes fear, but for other people climbing trees is fun!

So we can start to see that what we put on this graph is what we feel *not* what we are told to feel. If we 'feel' it is traumatic then that's good enough for this graph, it goes on! So you can see that climbing trees is 'subjective' as to whether it causes any fear or not.

So now let's move on by drawing 2 more memories that are traumatic represented by 3 blocks on the graph. I've drawn them here in BLUE. And now we are going to 'grade them' on a scale of 0 to 10, one being the lowest and ten being the highest.

We can explain "perhaps climbing the tree and feeling scared was a '5' on the scale when we think about it, and perhaps the other two blocks or memories (whatever they are you don't have to name them) are a '1', '3' and '10', that's a very bad one!" So now we have 'graded them' we have measured how much they affect us in UNITS.

We can draw the blocks similar in size to the number they represent, so a '1' block is small, a '10' block is large and a '5' is in between. It's just a visual representation that helps explain how they accumulate or you can just draw as best you can the same size – it's not an art class!

So we now have our first SUD's, we can explain "the memories on this graph are sad memories not happy ones. See how the title SUD's is made up? Let's put those there on the graph."

And now we are going to draw a new very important magical line in RED. Draw this from left to right along the top.

You can now explain this line represents our 'Tolerance to Stress' and that this line moves up and down in relation to the building blocks of stress, when the blocks are low the line remains HIGH, as the blocks grow in size they pull the line DOWN, as if the line was being pulled down by a magnet at the top of the blocks.

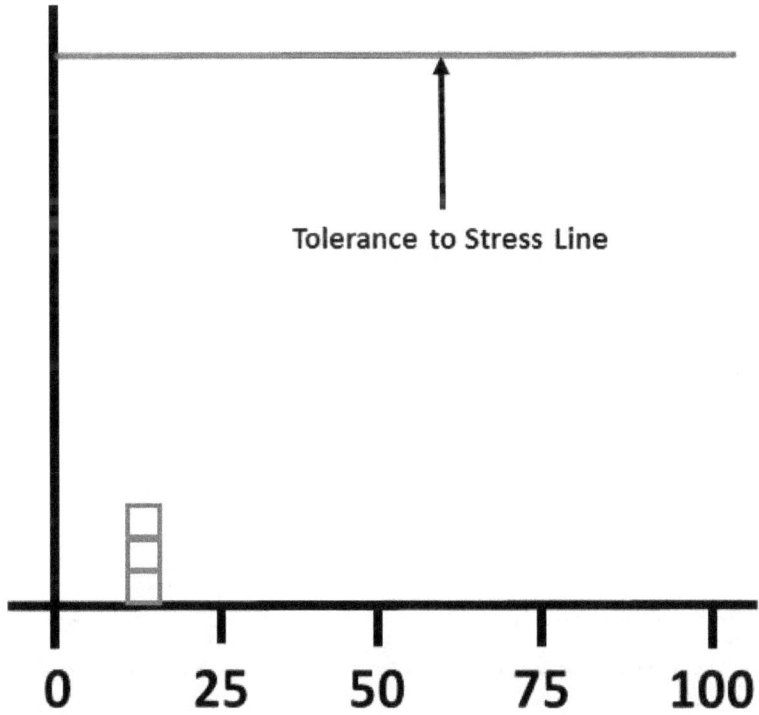

The red line moves down as our tolerance to stress REDUCES. I also sometimes add a reference to the red line as being the RED MIST that comes down, making our fuse shorter! Most people understand this once it's explained in this way! I place my pen horizontally hovering over and on the red line I've drawn and then move it up and down to simulate the line moving like this.

Let's go back to those four memories of those events or 'traumas'.

Our mind should almost immediately the moment the trauma happens start to process those events, like a conveyor belt. To demonstrate this I draw an arrow on the end of the base line to the right and use my pen to simulate the memory blocks moving along toward the end, "chug chug chug chug…"

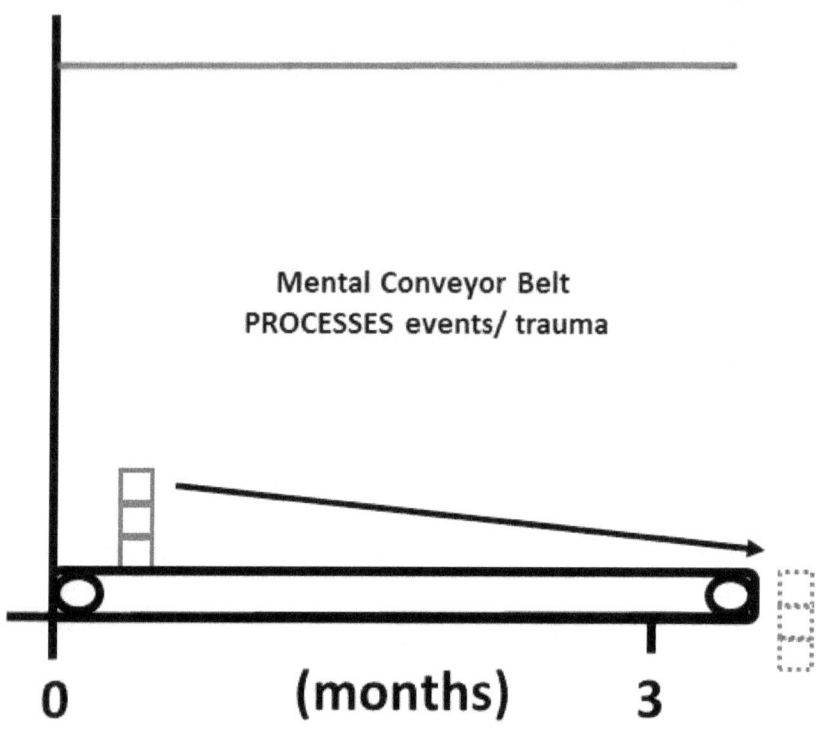

We can then go on to explain "the memories move along (chug chug chug chug as they go) and finally drop off the end". Explain "that might take 1 minute, 1 hour, 1 day, 1 week 1 month, but if it takes longer than 3 months – and after this magical time frame, the memory will become 'locked in'."

Now we can draw another helpful shape on the graph. If you imagine that this graph is going to end up in 3 sections, everything we are drawing here we are going to draw again two more times a bit further up the chart. So let's finish this first section by now drawing freehand in RED, a tall thin oval shape.

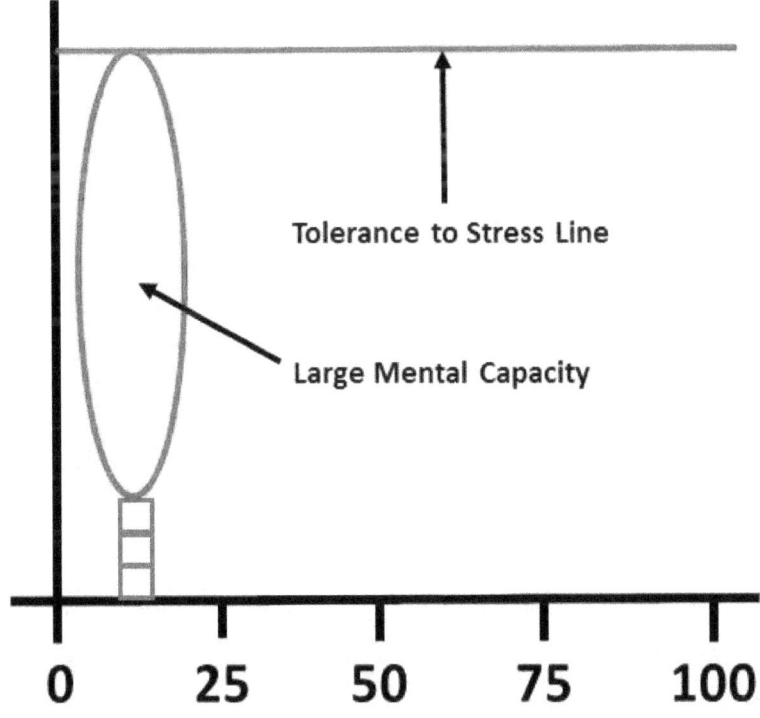

The top should touch the top horizontal RED line and the bottom should touch the top of the BLUE building blocks. I've drawn it adding it to the graph here for you to see. We're drawing this line because this shape – or space, represents just how much 'mental capacity' we have to deal with the everyday stress in our lives. It's a visual representation of our 'minds' space.

Explain "as you can see by the large size of the newly drawn RED oval there is a large amount of mental capacity, and that's why if the total of the building blocks only add up to between 0 and 25, we feel no stress at all from these events. In this example we can add up the total of the building blocks which was: 3 + 5 + 10 = 18 – The total SUD value is 18. As this is below 25 then we won't feel any stress and therefore the memories of these events do not concern us or affect our behaviour."

As we know we should have been able to process these events, BUT if our mind is still developing in childhood or the events we have witnessed are so traumatic we just can't make sense of them or let them go, then they stay ON our conveyor belt and DON'T drop off the end. OR if we are still trying to process them 3 months or more later on then the same thing happens.

It's like a hook appears and holds onto the memory. This 'memory hook' is how the mind remembers detailed memories and as such the memory cannot move into the subconscious mind, it stays put in our CONSCIOUS mind.

This is why we continue to experience, see, feel and witness the memory over and over again, it's called RUMINATION where we just keep going over the same thing again and again.

What happens then in this simple analogy is the start of the problem, or the point where the mind STOPS processing traumas. Our conveyor belt just stops!

All the building blocks now start to mount up even more and we start to feel 'weighted down' physically feeling the weight of our troubles on our mind. Clients are always very receptive to this explanation as they feel this.

Now as we move on to the next section of the graph, we just draw more blocks representing more life events that cause us trauma, about the same height again, so the size of the BLUE tower has now doubled.

As the tower grows the magnetic attraction, as it gets closer to the RED line, pulls the RED line DOWN again, and we can now draw that line on from left to right about 1cm lower than the previous line from the edge of the first larger red oval. We can explain "our TOLEREANCE to STRESS is now reducing".

As stress from more life events doubles or goes up by half again, the second RED oval (we can now draw) shows the mental capacity has DECREASED by half.

The stress has increased by half and the line has come down by half. The oval looks half the size so this appears to be perfectly rationale and obvious. This explanation always seems reasonable to people.

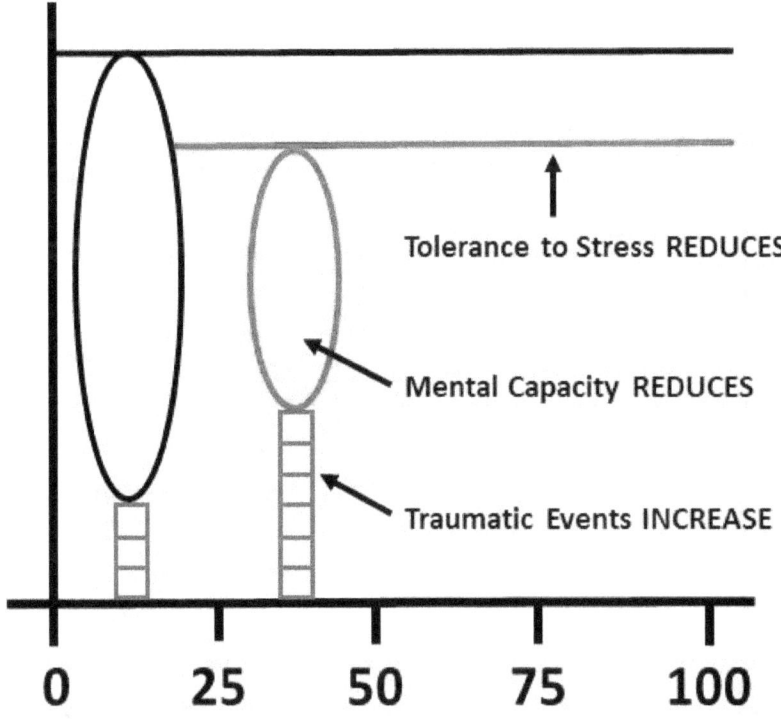

Now the accumulative total of the SUD's adds up to between 25 and 50, so we now feel generally stressed and when another life event then happens we feel and experience STRESS about that event.

Let's now add the final third section, as we now draw on even MORE blue building blocks of traumatic events, and now we will start to build and even ATTRACT more stressful events as our tower of stress now turns into a TOWER of ANXIETY.

Again we can now draw the blue blocks on at the same height again, so the size of the third BLUE tower has now increased by the same size again. As the tower grows now the magnetic attraction as it gets closer to the RED line once again now pulls the RED line DOWN.

We can now draw that line on from left to right about 1cm lower than the previous line from the edge of the second smaller red oval as we did twice before. We can explain again our TOLEREANCE to STRESS is now reducing significantly.

As the stress from more life events doubles again the RED oval we can now draw again shows the mental capacity has DECREASED by about a TWENTIETH of the size of the original oval, the stress has gone UP by HALF but it has reduced our mental capacity by far more than half, and that to all again feels about right.

We now feel restricted, closed in, finding it hard to cope and with what feels like no room to think – as can be demonstrated by the VERY SMALL RED OVAL we are finally left with. Now the final accumulative total of the SUD's adds up to between 50 and 75, we now no longer feel stressed about everything that is happening but, we now feel ANXIETY or anxious.

So when another event now happens we now feel and experience ANXIETY. This is a potentially dangerous place to be in, as if just one more building block of stress is added, as SOON AS it crosses our RED tolerance to stress line, we have a panic attack, a break down, we hide and run away or we lash out in RAGE completely bypassing anger altogether. Draw this on in RED. In this analogy the mind moves into a defensive state and puts the body into the 'Flight or Fight' mode permanently, the accumulation of stress moves directly to 100 instantly. It feels like it's the smallest but final straw.

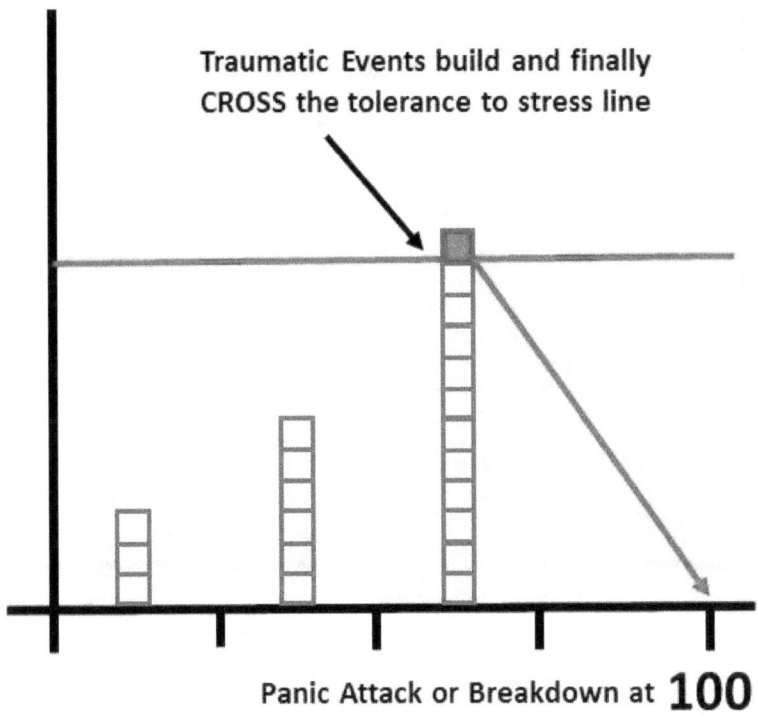

Now if the level of traumas keep building to over 100, we now see the feelings of ANXIETY develop into actual PHYSICAL conditions, like IBS, PAIN, SPASMS, which is why ANXIETY can cause Fibromyalgia, Chronic Pain Disorders, physical shaking and moving around that is highly noticeable. In fact there are a whole list of questions contained in a helpful questionnaire called the GAD7 test for Anxiety. There is another test for Depression – the PHQ-9 Test. You can find these self-diagnosis tests at the end of the book to take to see where you or your subject might be.

What happens next can be quite daunting for people. As our mind feels so TRAPPED by that RED line bearing down on us it doesn't like it, it recognises the danger we are in, and so it tries to RAISE THE LINE, to give us more mental capacity to function, by DISTRACTING US!

You can explain "DISTRACTIONS are almost an anagram of ADDICTIONS. We develop these distractions, addictive behaviours or actual addictions as a defence mechanism to try and cope or to forget about the traumas, to distract us from the anxiety. The mind does this because it is trying to RAISE or increase our tolerance to stress line, rather than by processing the trauma which it cannot any more as it's locked in."

These addictions appear to help us cope as we perhaps turn to:

- Smoking
- Alcohol
- Drugs
- Eating
- Gambling
- Shopping
- Self-Harm
- Cleaning
- Gaming

We call it the OVER BLANK game: What do you OVER ....?

OVER DRINK, OVER EAT, OVER BET, OVER SHOP, OVER...

As this is predominantly a book for children I have intentionally left out the areas that discuss in great detail all the 'Addictions' and how to treat them with EMDR. If you feel you or someone you know might benefit from this further highly detailed information I can recommend the EASY EMDR for Adults book, part of the set of nine titles in this series, or EASY EMDR for Addictions & OCD. Be aware children can also develop addictions like gaming and gambling.

There is another way of raising our tolerance to stress and that is with prescription medications, like anti-anxiety and anti-depressants. They act in the same way by chemically distracting our mind which increases our tolerance and so we can deal with everyday life better.

There are many other therapies that can also raise the 'tolerance to stress line' like CBT, Writing, Mindfulness, Yoga, Meditation, Art, Gardening the list goes on, but they only raise the line as long as you keep taking the medication or perform the therapy! So when you stop these the triggers, the causes of anxiety are still there!

Whilst taking prescription medication which can be very helpful for anyone with a dangerously reduced mental capacity, the level of mental capacity increases, which is why they are prescribed, but they do not fix the actual issues. The same goes for therapies that are undertaken before EMDR, they increase mental capacity but it has to be done daily else they fail and it's only a temporary fix.

So how does EMDR actually PERMANENTLY reduce and resolve anxiety and addictions, or treat PTSD or the associated disorders?

Quite simply by targeting the 'triggers' or the root causes of the memories of the traumas, we REDUCE the BLUE TOWER of ANXIETY, we turn DOWN the sensitivity of each block and continue to do that for each and every memory of trauma.

We then work on the other traumas until they have been resolved and the accumulative total of the SUD's is once again below 25. What then happens is the RED LINE, our tolerance to stress raises on its own as you can see in the graph below.

What I do to illustrate this is to simply squiggle out the big BLUE tower and explain "as the effect on memories reduce, or we become DESENSITISED to them (that's the D in EMDR), then the feelings of anxiety reduce, and we actually see this there and then in the same session!"

We start to even feel very much LIGHTER, often a very common reported experience by clients, as our mind begins to process events again and a weight is lifted off our mind literally, as we return to NORMAL levels.

Without the need for medication or therapy or addictions or distractions the amount of mental capacity now increases naturally without side effects.

Now rather than having what we have called POST TRAUMATIC STRESS we now enter a positive period of what can now be called:

POST TRAUMATIC GROWTH!

This is an incredible place to be, for some. It comes with its challenges. For people to go from having all these memories in their head and disturbing thoughts and feelings to now near nothing, it can feel empty, just like a blank canvas, ready to be filled with colour and images of new or older more familiar wonderful memories.

It can be often described as feeling as if the dark clouds have moved away revealing blue sky, or like a heavy physical weight literally being lifted. This can be a time for people to capitalise on their new found energy and mental strength, where people can literally go from strength to strength, being able to achieve far more than they had ever dreamed or thought possible.

For some people it means they can function after losing a loved one, return to work, come off benefits, perhaps just be able to go out of the house into public places or to a social situation is growth enough.

For other people it has meant they have had the strength to leave the refuge that has kept them safe and go back out into the wider world, with the support of other services, to set up home, and for some it has even meant the difference between loosing and keeping their children in the family court. Such is the power of EMDR it can truly help people who were once seen as sufferers to become achievers.

Here is a testimony from one such person below whose identity is validated but removed to maintain confidentiality. The words are powerful, strong, the direct opposite of when we first met:

"Since my first EMDR session I now feel less stressed, less emotional, less worried, less scared. I don't feel so anxious and I feel like a weight has been lifted as I don't feel so worried. Instead I now feel more confident in myself, I don't feel so frustrated with my son as I did before and I have noticed as a result of this he is calmer in himself and towards me. My sleep is deeper and longer as I'm less stressed. **The graph was very helpful explaining the treatment.**"

"Since my second EMDR session I feel amazing about myself, even more confident, more focused on things that I need to achieve in life. I now know I can do these things which is working in women's refuges to help other families. I don't feel so emotional, I feel level headed. Time with the kids is more relaxed, everything just seems easier and I'm actually wanting to go and take my kids and do things with them, without the worries of something happening. I'm not bothered about what others now have to say. My kids now say "you don't moan now mum"."

"I think that EMDR is brilliant, it's amazing. There should be more access to it. It should be put out there more. It should be promoted more. EMDR has got rid of all the crap in 2 sessions it's gone! It's proved to me it's worked 100% and I would highly recommend it."

Miss E - 2017

Chapter 6

Understanding the Basics of EMDR

So how does EMDR actually work? In order to understand what you are going to learn and how to practice it at home, it's best to first understand in simple terms how a therapist would carry out this treatment. Once you have a basic understanding of the treatment and how it's administered it's going to help you learn how to do exactly the same at home, quickly and easily!

All therapists operate differently, some require you to talk, others prefer a non-verbal approach using more advanced therapies. This is how I practice.

During the initial contact face to face or by phone, the EMDR therapist would ask you about your history, including what kind of symptoms or distress you are experiencing, whether or not you are taking any medication, have any addictions or OCD's, and what kind of support you are already receiving. Getting to know you in this way would help your therapist determine the best course of treatment.

If you're at home treating someone you already know, then you will already be fully aware of their history and this phase just isn't relevant, making treatment at home entirely possible, just as effective and actually it's therefore easier, which is why Home EMDR is faster!

Before EMDR treatment begins, your therapist would talk you through the second phase of the Theory and Discovery, by asking and answering any questions you may have. Eye Movement would be tested. All you would have to do is follow the therapist's fingers as they track across your eyesight line left and right.

At this point your therapist would relax you with simple breathing techniques, then work with you to recover all the memories and distressing locked in thoughts within your mind, like unravelling a ball of rubber bands.

In my clinic this is **MEMORY MAPPING**. The process is completely non-verbal (it's not counselling) allowing you to safely and quickly label (in the circles you will draw in front of you) any and all events that have caused you fear or feelings of shame or guilt.

EMDR is unique in that it can be non-verbal throughout and therefore suitable for many conditions such as Dyslexia, ADD, ADHD and Asperger's, and particularly children who would find it hard to express feelings about abuse, loss, stress & anxiety. It is also particularly good for adolescent boys, girls or often 'alpha' males who feel they cannot open up their emotions to a therapist.

I have worked with many such men and rather than entering into therapy I reframe the session as if we were in a gym or boxing ring (and often I do actually work with them in gyms and boxing rings) - we instead work on Strengthening and Conditioning the Mind! It's FITNESS for the MIND hence the adult version of this therapy is sometimes called MINDFIT.

As clients need not even divulge any information they can safely maintain their self-respect and work on issue A, B or C – as long as they in their own mind know what A relates to – perhaps Abuse, or B Bullying or Car crash or D Drugs, it doesn't affect the outcome of the therapy. In fact it enhances it as secrets can be safely resolved! This is why EMDR is so powerful as no secrets are sustained!

All the distressing thoughts and memories are written into circles that are then grouped where needed. Once the mind has been mapped your therapist would work with you to grade each memory on a scale of 1-10 of how distressing the memory is. This is the MEMORY MAPPING.

At this the third phase, you would now target the specific distressing memories identified in the MEMORY MAPPING phase with the eye movements.

To start with you would be asked to select an image to represent the event and then to focus on the amount of distress you feel and where you feel it in your body. This isolates and reconfirms the level of anxiety. Your therapist may help you to focus further with imaginative therapies if needed to ensure the feelings are those of anxiety.

Then your therapist would use bilateral eye movements until your distress has cleared (or is reduced as much as possible) and you are experiencing more positive thoughts and feelings and far less or even no anxiety at all! The process is then repeated again until all the issues are resolved in that same or subsequent sessions. A competent therapist would be able to treat 10-15 separate memories of trauma in just 1 session, reducing overall treatment time and cost.

The fourth phase is Re-evaluation which will take place in the session and is effectively the first step in your next session – if needed. This phase would see you and your therapist working together to consider how you are coping and whether or not you need to address the same memory as last time, or if you are able to move on to something different. It's important to recognise some people only need one session, for a significant number of multiple traumas you may need a few more than one session. At this stage it's just not possible to tell.

The nature of EMDR means that after your session the treatment will continue to be active in your awareness for 48 hours.

This means the effects of the treatment will continue to work, deepening the desensitisation, the overall resolution and the new feelings of positivity and calmness.

While everyone is different, over a short period of time (24-48 hours) these feelings will generally become far less intense although many people say they feel a strong sense of relief immediately in or after their sessions. This is one of the unseen phenomenal benefits of EMDR where Post Traumatic Stress turns into Post Traumatic GROWTH, where positive behaviours emerge.

It is common to feel tired shortly after the treatment and you should ensure you have a safe place (more than often at home) to rest, and if required to allow yourself to sleep. This sleep can often be highly restful and deep, as the mind continues to heal. It is commonly reported subjects awake feeling refreshed and even more positive, however this may take the recommended 1 – 2 days.

EMDR is NOT considered a form of hypnosis (which is a therapy not a treatment) but often Clinical Hypnotherapy can be used highly effectively to facilitate EMDR in cases where traumatic memories exist but cannot be recalled. Often very disturbing experiences become 'locked in' but out of conscious thought when the mind enters a hypnoidal or dreamlike state at the time the trauma occurs.

These events cannot be mapped in the second phase but Clinical Hypnosis can safely access these very deep rooted subconscious memories in order to then resolve them with EMDR. Combining these powerful methods can achieve long lasting and deep rooted positive change. You will need to visit a specialist therapist in person if you feel you have no ability to recall any trauma but are still suffering the effects of anxiety and post-traumatic stress. This is why EMDR is rapidly becoming the clinician's choice of medical treatment for the swift effective resolution of mental health issues.

Chapter 7

The simple four step EMDR process

Here is an outline of the 4 steps of EASY EMDR. You can refer back to this at any time, once you have mastered the breakdown of each step. Later on I'm going to breakdown each action fully with explanations and practical guidance of how to carry out the steps, with invaluable hints and tips on how to make the process easier, simpler and we are also going to look at what to not do. The guides are designed to repeat and overlap to aid learning and practical recall.

Each pf the three sections will relate to treating an adult, or an older or younger child and will explain how these differ. The adult explanation will always be provided first so you understand the full method and the children's versions will follow, so you can compare the difference and see how we use MAGIC to heal a child's MIND.

The first step you will see is **MEMORY MAPPING**, or **MIND MAGIC** which is the child version. There's a whole section on how to learn and use these simple techniques, here I'm just outlining the basic 4 steps of EMDR. I've covered all this in a lot more detail in the specific chapters to follow. This is just a quick outline, in a little more detail than the single trauma process, for information purposes just to show you how short the process is. It's going to be repeated and explained when I teach you how to use this for multiple trauma.

THE 4 STEPS for ADULTS

Step 1 – FIND

1. Identify traumatic memories by **MEMORY MAPPING**.
2. Grade Memory level from 1-10, Delete all under 5.
3. Group remaining memories if linked with lines.

Step 2 - FEEL

1. Close eyes - relax with breathing technique.
2. Focus on one memory group.
3. Increase memory emotion.
4. Isolate location of anxiety in body.
5. Recheck the level of anxiety (see Step 2).

Step 3 - FOLLOW

1. Open eyes focus on moving fingers left to right.
2. Ensure Eyes track fully left & right continuous.
3. Remind to focus on old memory & old feeling.
4. Feeling will subside. Memory will lessen.
5. Ask what level is desired 0, 1 or 2.
6. Check in with where the memory is.
7. Keep moving fingers/eyes erasing memory.
8. Memory will fade down to 2, 1, 0 gone (or the number chosen).

Step 4 - FORGET

1. Close eyes. Open eyes and answer break state questions.

2. After confusion reached close eyes.

3. Recheck memory. If gone end. Move to next group.

4. If not gone has feeling gone? End. Move to next group.

5. If memory and feeling present - grade (go to Step 3).

So now we have an understanding of how the process works for adults, overleaf is an outline of the basic steps for Older Children, which are the same as for adults except we use magic to make the therapy fun and engaging and I've covered all this in a lot more detail in the chapters to come.

I've then outlined the basic process for younger children using FINGER PUPPETS, which again we will cover in far more detail in the specific chapters that follow.

THE 4 STEPS for Older Children – using MIND MAGIC

Step 1 – FIND

1. Show the child the magical illustrations.

2. Use wand to pull out memory and place into a bottle.

3. Ask child to label the bottle. They have now effectively labelled the memory.

Step 2 – FEEL

4. Pour the memory into the Magic Circle or Crystal Ball - draw a circle and write the name from the bottle in the circle.

5. Ask child to focus on the memory and close eyes keep focusing on memory.

6. Ask how bad the memory is on a scale of 1-10.

7. Ask where can they 'feel' the memory. Once the feeling is identified ask them to focus on the feeling and the memory.

Step 3 – FOLLOW

8. Ask the child to open their eyes and then use the wand to track eyes left and right. Memory reduces.

9. Close eyes. Open eyes break state with questions leading to confusion. Close eyes.

Step 4 – FORGET

10. Attempt to Re-trigger the memory. If not gone repeat eye tracking.

11. When 'gone' move to next memory begin process again.

THE 4 STEPS for Younger Children (with Finger Puppets)

Step 1 – FIND

1. Ask the child to choose one Finger Puppet from a selection.

   Use finger puppet or TheraPlay to identify the trauma (we will cover this in far greater detail later).

Step 2 – FEEL

2. Ask child to close eyes and keep focusing on memory.

3. Ask how bad the memory is using the arrow on the scale of 1-10.

4. Ask where can they 'feel' the memory. Once the feeling is identified ask them to focus on the feeling and the memory.

Step 3 – FOLLOW

5. Ask the child to open their eyes and then use the finger puppet to track eyes left and right. Memory reduces.

6. Close eyes. Open eyes break state with questions leading to confusion. Close eyes.

Step 4 – FORGET

7. Attempt to Re-trigger the memory. If not gone repeat eye tracking.

8. When 'gone' allow the child to go and play and reward, move to next memory after 2 days and begin process again.

After treatment

NB. Once memory has gone sleep will aid recovery in all age groups.

Adrian Radford-Shute DHP Acc. Hyp.

Chapter 8

Step 1 – 'FIND' for Adults

I'm going to explain here at the outset how all the stages are set out and how to learn from them. At first I'm going to explain the long version of what we are doing, why we are doing it, how it helps, and what to do with comments and tips, help and guidance. There are further simple illustrations to help found at Chapter 15.

At the end of each section I've written out the short version of EXACTLY what to say in the step by step guide or SCRIPT. I've then compiled ALL the guides together in a separate section of the book later on so you can refer to this and just follow the guide all the way through the entire session with ease.

I suggest you read this long version through once or twice, then practice reading out the session script on your own by yourself first so you get the hang of what to do, what actions to take and what to say at the right time. Once you are happy with the flow then practice on another person where possible if not use the subject.

Once you are confident which will only take just a few go's it's really very simple, then you will be proficient to work with a live subject.

Remember when you're working with a live subject you're just going to follow the short guide notes, found at Chapter 15, read out exactly what's written, nice and calmly with a mellow therapy or 'velvet' voice where possible. You can listen to how this should sound with practical demonstrations and tutorials at **www.EASYEMDR.org**.

STEP 1 – FIND

In order to carry out the first step in the treatment process for stress or anxiety, we need to know what it is we are treating, so before we begin we need to identify what's not working, what needs attention, and what the cause is. It's the same as if taking a car to a garage with a fault for example:

The general issue is the car isn't running properly or not as it should do, it's making noises, its behaving differently etc. The garage first of all will need to carry out a diagnostic check to identify what's causing the problem.

Let's say the problem is there's smoke coming from the exhaust, the garage isn't going to fix the smoke by blocking up the exhaust - that would make it worse! The garage isn't going to run another pipe so you can't see the smoke – that's just a distraction – or a coping strategy! In order to FIX the problem the garage will need to run a computer diagnostic check, then look inside the engine, find out if it's a gasket, is it an injector, is it an oil leak, it may be all of them, and once they know they can then focus their work on fixing that part, then they will fix the next part and so on until the car is fully repaired.

They can't repair everything at once it's a process, and using EASY EMDR is no different! So we are going to run a check on the body's computer – the MIND! This process is MEMORY MAPPING. Then we are going to look at the report and find out which aspects we need to focus on to fix the mind. MEMORY MAPPING simply put is the exact same process, and it's simple. You certainly don't need any type of degree or medical experience to do this.

If you're working with adults you can start quite easily using the simple circle method below. This will allow you to work out the causes of anxiety, and once you've done this, then you'll use EMDR to treat what's in each circle later on. All the information needed comes from the subject hence there is no medical knowledge needed!

If you're working with older children the process is still simple, but you will need to use different language that they can identify with. This is one of the major difficulties therapists have when working with children and why it's so specialised, but thanks to the world of magic I've made this so simple it's highly effective and can be fun! If therapy with children is fun then they will engage with and trust in the process, you'll see the results you're hoping for.

If you are working with much younger children who wouldn't understand magic or the concept of spells, then we can use another simple fun system with finger puppets and art. It will take a little longer but the results will be the same, a little more patience and dedication may be required but it still can be fun and very rewarding for the younger child and indeed the parent.

It's best to learn the simple adult version first, its quick and easy and once mastered you can then add in the elements needed to make it age appropriate for children by introducing the magical spells, or the finger puppets and art.

This unique process is the system by which EMDR can be safely accelerated to achieve results, as often seen in the very same session.

This process is absolutely key and central to the effective treatment of anxiety and EMDR, its important you understand this section before moving on. It takes very little effort to achieve such an incredible outcome. Clients always describe this process as being very helpful, almost calming in itself and quite mindful – it allows the person to understand what's been causing their anxiety, their anger, their changes in behaviour, their addictions, and or their sadness.

Once it has been drawn the healing process has already begun!

MEMORY MAPPING FOR ADULTS

The Basics

The AIM of this section, the first stage, is to teach and demonstrate to you:

- How to relax your subject
- How to draw the circles to aid MEMORY MAPPING
- What to remember
- How and what to write
- How to grade the memories
- How to delete unnecessary memories
- How to group the remaining memories

Once this has been completed you will then have developed the all-important TREATMENT PLAN - a guide to how many sessions needed and what to do first.

The OBJECTIVE of this stage is to build TRUST in the process and to UNJUMBLE the mind, as you will then follow this plan or Memory Map when you carry out the EASY EMDR treatment. These then become your 'home clinic notes'.

If you imagine the confused mind is like a ball of rubber bands and each band is a distressing memory, thought or feeling, when we look at the ball we can't make sense of what is what. That's pretty much how most people are going to feel if they have experienced MULTIPLE TRAUMA.

Multiple Trauma is where someone has experienced more than one episode or memory of trauma that are unconnected. For people who only have one SINGLE TRAUMA this section is straightforward and actually very easy.

Let's say someone had a car accident and we are going to use EASY EMDR to help their mind recover, all we need to work on is the one subject – CAR ACCIDENT. The mind isn't confused it's very clear on what the distressing image or memory is and we can start almost start straight away with that.

But if there are years of MULTIPLE TRAUMA or distressing memories and now distressing thoughts have taken hold, it may be hard for the person to identify all the causes. It's very common and often in therapy this is what takes up so much session time, but with this unique system of MEMORY MAPPING we can unjumble the ball of rubber of bands, one by one relatively quickly! When all the bands are separated the person can then see what distressing thoughts have made up their ball of stress. Once we have this we can work on each band – that's actually a memory, thought or feeling.

Unjumbling the Mind

When we first start this process our subject is going to feel anything from a little apprehensive to perhaps experiencing increased anxiety, this is usual. The process here will start to calm the mind, and as it does so calm the senses that then seem to close off. This allows the subject to focus deeper on the memories, which simply put is unjumbling the mind and making sense of their thoughts and fears as their intuition takes over helping them to 'pull out' everything.

We can help our subject calm their mind from this initial anxiety by simply asking them to breathe in the following way:

Ask your subject to close their eyes and breathe IN for FOUR (that's counting to 4 slowly).

Say "BREATHE IN FOR 4 FILLING YOUR LUNGS & SHOULDERS" perhaps you can do it with them to demonstrate as they breathe in – I always do as it helps create and establish the trust that you're going to be there and help them all the way.

Once they have breathed in for four seconds ask them to "HOLD IT HOLD IT" and they will gently hold their breath.

Then immediately ask them to breathe OUT for EIGHT (that's counting to 8 very slowly NOT 8 seconds it may take around 16 seconds) breathing all the air out – again I do this with them making a noise while exhaling to simply demonstrate how to slowly and calmly exhale all the air in the lungs.

Repeat this again asking them to breathe IN for FOUR filling the lungs and shoulders and HOLD IT, HOLD IT then breathe OUT again for EIGHT.

Repeat one last time – IN FOR FOUR, HOLD IT, HOLD IT, AND BREATHE OUT FOR EIGHT.

Your subject will now feel calmer. The reason why this technique is so valuable is medically evidenced. When we feel threatened or frightened a chemical called CORTISOL is released from our brain, this triggers ADRENALIN which is pumped around our body rapidly by our heart rate increasing. The adrenalin fires into the muscles into our legs and arms so our strength increases temporarily which gives us the ability to run away faster – it's a survival reaction – the infamous 'Fight or Flight' response, as we've discussed earlier. This adrenalin is the cause of the feeling of anxiety! So if we slow the heart rate when cortisol is triggered because we are frightened or feeling anxious, then less adrenalin is pumped around the body and the anxiety therefore decreases.

It's a highly simple yet highly effective breathing technique that will calm people in moments of stress or distress. You can use this at any time if you're feeling anxious or stressed, not just with EASY EMDR! Go ahead and try it yourself now speaking all the words on the next page out loud:

1. CLOSE YOUR EYES
2. BREATHE IN FOR 4 FILLNG YOUR LUNGS AND SHOULDERS
3. HOLD IT... HOLD IT...
4. BREATHE OUT SLOWLY FOR 8 EXHALE ALL THE AIR
5. BREATHE IN FOR 4 FILLING YOUR LUNGS AND SHOULDERS
6. HOLD IT... HOLD IT...
7. BREATHE OUT SLOWLY FOR 8 EXHALE ALL THE AIR
8. BREATHE IN FOR 4 FILLING YOUR LUNGS AND SHOULDERS
9. HOLD IT... HOLD IT... HOLD IT
10. BREATHE OUT SLOWLY FOR 8 EXHALE ALL THE AIR
11. OPEN YOUR EYES FEELING SO MUCH MORE RELAXED

With practice this simple exercise can slow your rate of breath to just TWO breaths a minute! If it takes 10 seconds to breathe in for FOUR and HOLD and 20 seconds to breathe out and relax that's 30 seconds – certainly enough to slow even the most anxious person's heart rate – and it's only breathing!

We are going to use this breathing technique a lot during the EASY EMDR process as it's very helpful in keeping our subjects calm and it can be used by adults and children of all ages.

By calming the heart we also start to calm the mind as we have also lowered our subject's brainwave activity. This is important for EMDR because simply put the lower the brainwave activity the calmer we become and as a result the more focused we become on what's deep inside our mind as our other senses seem to turn off and our 'intuition' comes to the fore.

This helps us with the MEMORY MAPPING process as when we engage with our subconscious mind it helps us to draw out or recover the memories of what is actually causing the anxiety deep down inside.

My clients often tell me when we first speak that they have no idea of what's causing their anxiety, but after this process they can clearly see exactly what the causes are and straight away they begin to feel so much better already. Because now they know, and they have now made good progress already!

Now unless you're a therapist, clinician, medical professional or someone wanting to gain a much deeper understanding of EMDR, or perhaps you're interested in a career as a therapist, then you won't need to learn about brainwave activity, but if you are interested I've included all this information in the EASY EMDR Professional book.

Drawing the Circles

Now our subject is calm we can begin to draw the all-important 'circles':

1. Place a few pieces of A4 paper landscape on a clip board. Use a black or blue pen. Keep hold of the clip board you are just demonstrating at this time.

2. YOU draw a medium sized circle in the top left corner about the size of a ping pong ball about 5cm across. This demonstrates what the subject should do to follow.

3. Explain to the subject that in a minute they are going to write just ONE or TWO words in that circle.

4. Explain to the subject not to worry about what to write just yet as you are going to cover this in more detail in a moment (see below).

5. Explain to the subject once they have written in the circle they will then draw another same size circle to the right of the first circle next to the first one.

6. Explain to the subject to then focus on the blank circle they have just drawn. Explain to the subject by doing this the subject will not be focusing on what they've just written and will not feel the anxiety related to the memory they have just described.

7. Invite the subject to again write just ONE or TWO words in that circle.

8. Keep repeating the exercise again and again drawing circles and writing words until the subject knows when to STOP, which is covered below.

9. If the subject doesn't draw a circle simply ASK them quietly to 'DRAW A CIRCLE' and point to the place where the circle should be drawn, remind them to FOCUS on the BLANK CIRLCE they have just drawn, NOT dwell on what they have just written. It's up to YOU to keep the process flowing, don't let them stop other than to focus on a blank circle – until they have finished of course.

It's important to explain to the subject that it's not a competition, some people draw only one circle because they have only one SINGLE issue or trauma they need to deal with, other people may draw 4 circles, or 10, 20 or even 40 or more.

This is why you need a few sheets of paper on your clipboard as you don't want to run out interrupting the flow.

What to Write

Each circle acts as a LABEL for a memory. That's all it is. It's a visual representation of a distressing memory, thought or feeling. You can think of each circle as a snapshot image, like a Polaroid photo that's been named. All we are looking for to be written in each circle is just ONE or TWO words as a label or name to describe that photo, or snapshot image, that memory.

Here's a few examples:

TRAUMATIC MEMORY = I fell out of a Cherry Tree.

LABEL = TREE or CHERRY TREE or FALL or ACCIDENT

To us the 'home therapist' it doesn't matter what the words are, the only person they must matter to is the Subject! As long as when you say "We are now going to work on CHERRY TREE" the subject knows what that memory is connected too, then that is all we need – simple!

The subject may feel that if however they write a word that can be easily be recognised and cause embarrassment or an issue by disclosing something they are not confident to, they can abbreviate or choose a simple code word. Here's a few examples:

TRAUMATIC MEMORY = Sexually Abused

LABEL = BATHROOM or 'A' or ORANGE

We as the 'home therapist' or family member may not know what these words relate to, they could mean anything, but to the subject the label 'A' or BATHROOM is perhaps where the abuse happened or the initial of the word 'Abused' or perhaps ORANGE was the colour of a towel etc.

This is why the EASY EMDR process must be NON VERBAL so that the subject will NEVER need to explain or discuss or elaborate on what the meaning of the word is as that could be a barrier to engaging in treatment.

It's important to understand and explain to the subject that firstly what they write is CONFIDENTIAL to them, we do not need to know! Second it's technically none of our business, we are there to help them heal not to enter into counselling – as we know this rarely actually resolves locked in trauma!

With this unique approach it's safe for a family member, friend or colleague to work with someone very close to them, which is very rare in any type of therapy. This is why EASY EMDR and this unique Memory Mapping process is probably so incredible, ground breaking and ultimately most helpful.

As the 'home therapist' you must NEVER ask anyone to explain what they have written, but if they choose to speak just listen and do NOT comment, although allowing people to speak will just slow down the process. EMDR is mainly non-verbal and it isn't required.

Some people will have difficulty writing, perhaps they are too young, dyslexic or have lost use of their arm due to injury. It's ok to ask them what they would like to call the circle and then you can write it down for them. If the subject prefers to write their own words but you cannot read their writing or their spelling is not proficient it doesn't matter at all, you can just ask them when the time comes "what does this say?" instead.

In order to keep the process flowing usually we do not need to intervene, we just quietly ask or remind the subject to "WRITE WHAT COMES INTO YOUR MIND", they do so, then draw another circle and label it – great! If they pause on an empty circle just ask the subject again calmly to "WRITE WHAT COMES INTO YOUR MIND", they do so, then draw another circle and write again. If they pause on drawing a circle you can remind them to "DRAW ANOTHER CIRCLE, FOCUS ON THE CIRCLE AND WRITE WHAT COMES INTO YOUR MIND".

If the Subject becomes 'Stuck'

Now we've just said we shouldn't intervene and that's right, as we are allowing the subject to unjumble their own mind, memory by memory, and as one memory is written down the mind will deepen and allow access to another memory, and the mind will keep going deeper and deeper.

If the subject however is stuck we can now intervene safely and help them indirectly or directly, which is responsible, and here's how:

If they are STUCK and they will say this or just stop writing, it means there is a memory there but they either can't access it clearly or they are having trouble labelling it. Now we just revert back to the breathing exercise we carried out at the start of the session. Nearly everyone gets stuck so this is why we practice the breathing at the beginning to calm the subject but also to teach them what to do during MEMORY MAPPING. It should start to all be making sense now!

So if the subject is stuck, ask them to close their eyes as we've done before and:

1. BREATHE IN FILLING YOUR LUNGS AND SHOULDERS
2. HOLD IT... HOLD IT...
3. BREATHE OUT SLOWLY EXHALE ALL THE AIR
4. BREATHE IN FILLING YOUR LUNGS AND SHOULDERS
5. HOLD IT... HOLD IT..
6. BREATHE OUT SLOWLY EXHALE ALL THE AIR
7. BREATHE IN FILLING YOUR LUNGS AND SHOULDERS
8. HOLD IT... HOLD IT... HOLD IT (an extra hold is needed)
9. BREATHE OUT SLOWLY EXHALE ALL THE AIR
10. WITH YOUR EYES CLOSED CONTINUE TO BREATHE NORMALY
11. IN A MOMENT I'M GOING TO ASK YOU TO OPEN YOUR EYES, WHEN I DO FOCUS SOFTLY ON THE CIRCLE YOU'VE JUST DRAWN AND WRITE WHAT COMES INTO YOUR MIND
12. OPEN YOUR EYES AND WRITE WHAT COMES INTO YOUR MIND

The subject will then start to write again and the process continues.

If they become stuck again further on, simply ask the subject to close their eyes and instruct them in the breathing exercise all over again.

Using this simple technique will allow blocks to be removed and the subject will go deeper and deeper into their own mind, pulling out often very deep rooted memories.

This process calms the mind even further, it turns off other senses and the mind just focuses on what it needs to remember, this is how we help subjects recover memories they couldn't find or had blocked.

Because at this stage the mind has entered a very calm brain cycle the THETA cycle (you can read more about this in the Professional version of EASY EMDR if you wish) true memories and feelings are revealed. Often the subject when asked had no idea they were holding onto that memory, but it's there!

Knowing when to stop

At some point the subject will just stop and they will categorically KNOW they have finished. It's a very different feeling and body language to someone who is 'stuck'. Once they have finished you can move onto the next step, but only after you've checked everything they need to cover is recorded in one of the circles.

To do this simply ask the subject "As you now look over everything that you've remembered is there anything you can remember that you've left out, is there anything else you'd like to add or work on?".

That question will lead to two possible answers; NO or YES, and if it's a YES simply ask the subject to draw another circle and label that memory. Remember to ask the same question again! Don't assume there was only one memory left!

What we have covered here is an INDIRECT approach where the subject directs the therapy and brings forward what they are happy to work on, this is always the best approach to start.

However, if you are working with a family member or friend and you know some of the person's history and you are concerned they haven't addressed the issues you discussed, then you can change the approach to become DIRECTED by you.

All this means is you now DIRECT the therapy and to do this you can simply ask them directly "Is the issue (you can name the subject matter) we discussed written here?" Again the subject will answer YES and probably show you (they may have described or labelled the memory in a different way to what you were expecting – see the CHERRY TREE example below), or NO, again ask them to draw a circle and label that memory.

If they chose not to you must respect that decision and do not push the subject or they will simply not engage in the process. Perhaps come back to the circle when they feel more comfortable and just work with what you have gathered at that time.

Grading the Memories

Once all the circles have been drawn we now need to GRADE them. For this use a RED pen, it helps create stand out from all the detail.

We ask the subject to GRADE the memories by writing a number in each circle from 0 – 10. Explain to the subject to FEEL the number not THINK. Explain to the subject their mind will intuitively know what the number is. Explain to the subject 0 is low and 10 is high. Explain to the subject this number represents how 'bothered' they are by what's written in the circle, or how painful it feels, or how distressing the memory is. We learnt about Subject Units of Distress before, well this is the UNIT part.

The subject will start to write a number in each circle in RED, instruct them to just move straight onto the next circle and just keep going and not to dwell, just write what number comes into their mind.

This is a relatively easy process for 100% of all clients I have ever treated. Grading the numbers happens almost fluidly.

At the end of the process (or even tot them up as they go along if you want to appear to be smart and very good at Math!) add up the numbers. They will give you a total of perhaps 34, or 56, or 79 or 98 – anything up to 100 is very common. However in some cases I've had clients go over to 136 or 224 even up to over 360 which is not common, one client was over 650 which is rare, but it's still ok, it just means they have experienced far more trauma than most (by the way they still only took 3 sessions of EMDR to fully resolve 684 units!).

Once you have the total you can refer them back to the ANXIETY GRAPH and show them where they sit on that chart. It's at this stage that often a moment of eureka happens as the subject for the first time realises why they feel the way they feel, because they can see it on the graph. It's so important to explain to them THIS is why they feel the way they do because of the accumulative effect of all the historical traumas they've gone through, which add up to a number which reflects how stressed or anxious they feel.

Remind them, a total score between 0-25 means they will not feel stressed, a score between 25-50 means they will feel stress, a score between 50-75 means they will be experiencing anxiety in their daily lives and their behaviours will start to change as the mind starts to distract it from the anxiety its feeling, and over 75 means they are suffering from acute anxiety.

But a high number does not necessarily mean they will need many EMDR sessions, as now we are going to work out which memories we actually need to work on which ones we can cross off!

This again speeds up the treatment process helping the subject to become healthful much quicker. This can also be a relief for the subject as it cuts down recovery time too – that's positive!

Deleting low grade Memories

We are now going to DELETE any memory graded 4 or lower by crossing them out with a RED line through the circle. We simply don't need to work on these as they do not cause sufficient anxiety to be of concern. Once the higher graded memories have been reprocessed the subjects mind will usually be able to process these lower grade traumas on their own.

Again this is how we can speed up the treatment process because as 'home therapists' we DON'T need to treat every low grade memory the subject has ever had, which again speeds up the treatment.

We can go even further and ask the subject, working through the circles line by line, if it's OK to cross out any memory graded lower than a 5. As a 5 is on the border line some memories can be deleted, perhaps others should stay and be worked on, and it's the subject's choice. If they are unsure KEEP the circle.

So again we can safely perhaps delete even more speeding up the process even more! This is why EASY EMDR is credible and ethical.

Grouping Memories

We are now going to speed up the process safely even further by GROUPING memories - where possible!

With EASY EMDR as a Specialist Practitioner I am able to work on more than one memory at a time and I'm going to share this knowledge with you too, so you can work at the same level! It's very simple and here's how:

Ask the subject if any of the memories happened at the same time, can they be grouped together? Use those exact words. Here's an example to use:

MEMORIES/LABELS WRITTEN IN THE CIRCLES:

1. CHERRY TREE
2. BREAKING LEGS
3. PAIN WALKING
4. CAR ACCIDENT
5. MOTHERS DEATH

As you can see we have 5 memories to carry out EASY EMDR on. Let's say on average it takes 5 minutes per memory that's 25 minutes. Now the subject says the first three are all connected, when they fell out of the CHERRY TREE they ended up BREAKING LEGS.

That went on to cause PAIN WALKING, so they are CONNECTED and can be GROUPED. So now draw a line between each circle joining them together, but the 4th and 5th memories are separate, they happened much later in the subjects life perhaps, so do NOT link these with a line. Let's take a look:

The memory map GROUPS will now look like this:

1. CHERRY TREE, BREAKING LEGS, PAIN WALKING
2. CAR ACCIDENT
3. MOTHERS DEATH

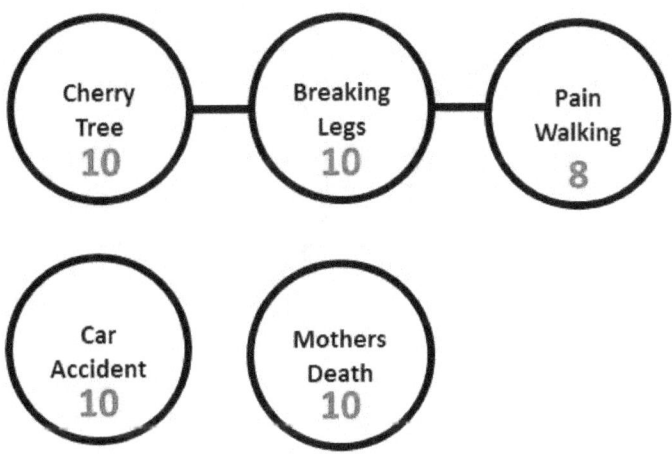

We now have 3 grouped memories to work on rather than 5 so the treatment time at 5 minutes per trauma is now only 15 minutes! You can see how grouping memories can speed up the EMDR treatment process rapidly and thus the healing time.

This is how I regularly treat clients who present with 20-60 traumatic memories at the same time in just a few sessions rather than the medical guidelines of 6-12 sessions.

When grouping you may find there are 5-10 circles grouped, just draw a line between each one connecting them all as a single string.

You may find that lines start to cross with multiple trauma MEMORY MAPS. If they do simply draw two very small straight lines like brackets or a map bridge symbol to record the direction of flow of lines that cross, like this where FC and Flower are connected and B & School are connected:

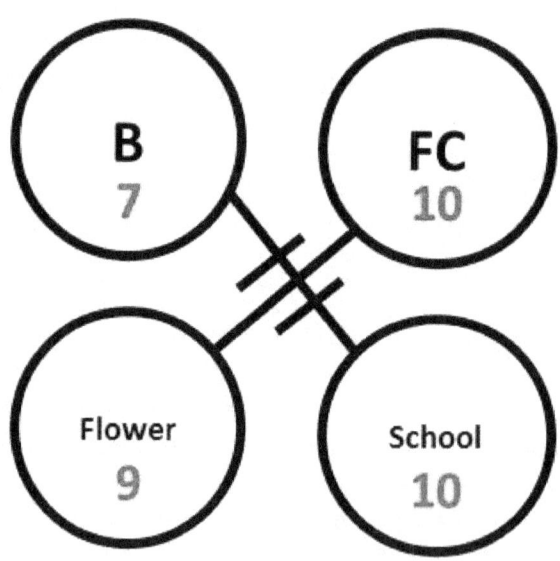

The finalised MEMORY MAP may now look like this example:

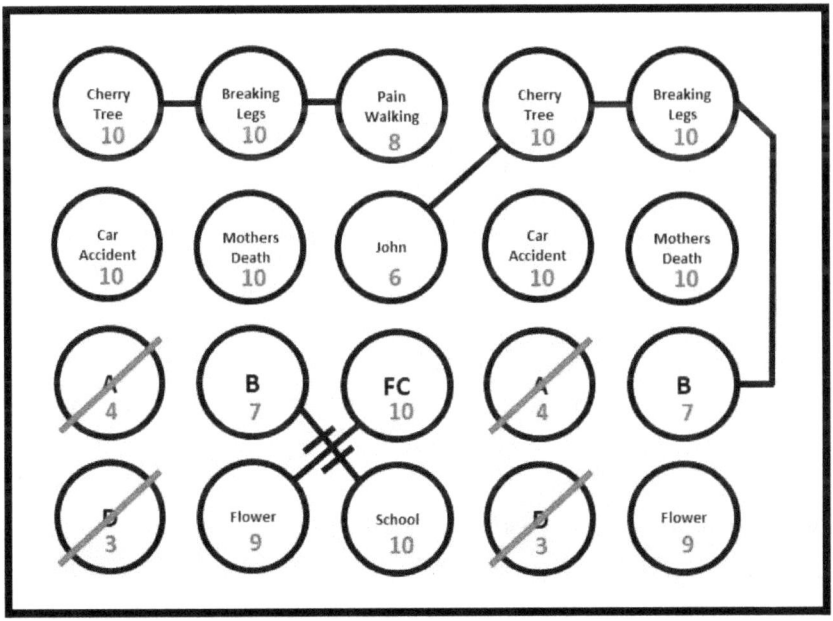

What if the subject becomes distressed during MEMORY MAPPING?

During the MEMORY MAPPING process it is unlikely, but still possible that your subject may become distressed in that they may become sad, feel anxious or even cry. This can seem frightening to anyone but it is important you remain focused and continue to guide the subject to draw the next circle etc. Often just this one action alone is enough to allow the subject to regain composure and carry on. Here's a good way of describing to someone this reaction or 'abreaction' as it is referred to clinically;

"Traumas can be like a Firework going off! Sometimes they just sparkle with a little bang, sometimes they go off with a big bang! But soon as they do they ALL start to fizzle out and disappear and once a Firework has been lit and has gone off it can never be re-lit again – it's finished! It's Gone!"

This is how EMDR works with even the most distressing of memories.

There can be very rare cases where a subject will not be able to carry on and may be overcome with emotion. When drawing the graph it will already become apparent very early on if your subject is likely to experience what may appear to be uncontrollable emotion, as your subject will already show signs of being very emotional from the outset and you will be more aware of the possibility of an abreaction.

In this instance, if you are aware this may happen it is important to distract the person from what they are feeling and we do this by simply taking them to a 'SAFE PLACE' in their mind. If your subject shows signs of heightened emotion from the outset then it would always be best to set this SAFE PLACE up before starting any of the MEMORY MAPPING process.

To set up a SAFE PLACE ask the subject to first identify and name a place they consider to be safe; their home, bedroom, holiday, beach, mountain top! It doesn't have to be safe to us, it is where they feel they can safely go to in their mind where no harm can come to them, a place where they are in control. Once they have named this place ask them to close their eyes and imagine being there. You can help them by asking them to describe the location, room, temperature, colours, what they can see, but importantly how they feel. Once you know they feel SAFE you can explain to them they can go back to this place whenever YOU instruct them too and they WILL be safe.

You can test this by asking the subject to describe what they were doing yesterday and after a little while interrupt the conversation sharply – immediately take control and firmly ask them to CLOSE THEIR EYES AND GO TO YOUR SAFE PLACE NOW! Once they are there ask them to describe it again and how they feel, it will be the same as before. Your subject now knows they can proceed safely.

So if during the MEMORY MAPPING process they become distressed enough that they cannot continue you MUST take control of the situation and instruct them firmly to CLOSE THEIR EYES AND GO TO YOUR SAFE PLACE NOW! Once they are there ask them to describe it again and how they feel, it will be the same as before. Your subject will begin to calm. Now use the 4 IN 8 OUT breathing technique the subject has already learnt.

You may then choose to continue with the process which is advisable, starting on a new blank circle. Remember you can always use this technique in the highly unlikely event your subject becomes overly distressed at any point.

It is important to only intervene where absolutely necessary, as if you do so every time the subject shows a little emotion you will never be able to target the actual trauma, and when we come on to do this it is very common that there is always some degree of distress, as we are recalling sad or upsetting memories not happy ones. There's lots more help on this later in the book.

No matter what you do they are already aware of the memories so you cannot make anything worse or bring up feelings that were hidden or repressed as they are already in the person's conscious memory. To do this you would need to use Clinical Hypnotherapy, which is why this book does NOT teach or explain the use of such regression processes as this kind of therapy should only be carried out by trained and experienced therapists in a clinical setting.

So now we know how in detail to carry out the MEMORY MAPPING for adults, we can now go on to practice this step. I've written out the exact wording to use for the entire phase of this part of the session – this is what we call a 'SCRIPT'. Once you become proficient enough in its contents you can do away with it, like a professional therapist would. It's just a guide to get you going, a synopsis of everything we've already covered before.

I've put together the entire scripts with illustrations for adults and children at Chapters 15, 16 & 17 for quick and easy reference titled "Conduct a Session for …..".

MEMORY MAPPING SCRIPT - ADULTS STEP 1 'FIND'

TO HELP YOU RESOLVE THE FEELINGS AND THOUGHTS AND ANXIETY YOU'VE BEEN HAVING I'M JUST GOING TO TALK YOU THROUGH THIS SIMPLE GRAPH SO WE UNDERSTAND WHY WE HAVE BEEN FEELING THE WAY DO, AND THIS GRAPH IS THEN GOING TO LEAD US ON TO IDENTIFYING THE CAUSES AND THAT'S WHAT WE ARE THEN GOING TO USE THE EMDR ON, TO RESOLVE THOSE FEELINGS AND MEMORIES.

(Explain and talk through the anxiety graph – a copy of which can be found at Chapter 5.)

SO NOW WE KNOW WHAT CAUSES THE ANXIETY WE NOW HAVE TO FIGURE OUT EXACTLY WHAT ALL THESE BUILDING BLOCKS ARE.

AND WE ARE GOING TO DO THAT BY DRAWING AND LABELLING SOME CIRCLES NICE AND EASY.

IT'S NOT A COMPETITION HOW MANY CIRCLES YOU DRAW, SOME PEOPLE DRAW ONLY ONE, OTHERS DRAW 4 CIRCLES, OR 10, 20, SOME PEOPLE DRAW 40 OR MORE IT DOESN'T MATTER.

EACH CIRCLE ACTS AS A LABEL FOR A DISTRESSING MEMORY. THAT'S ALL IT IS. THINK OF EACH CIRCLE AS A SNAPSHOT IMAGE, LIKE A POLAROID PHOTO THAT'S BEEN NAMED. ALL YOU NEED TO WRITE IN EACH CIRCLE IS JUST ONE OR TWO WORDS THAT LABEL OR NAME OR DESCRIBE THAT PHOTO, OR SNAPSHOT IMAGE OF THE MEMORY.

LET ME GIVE YOU AN EXAMPLE:

A TRAUMATIC MEMORY I HAVE IS FALLING OUT OF A CHERRY TREE.

SO THE LABEL I'M GOING TO WRITE COULD BE 'TREE' OR 'CHERRY TREE' OR 'FALL' OR 'ACCIDENT' – AS LONG AS YOU KNOW WHAT THE WORD RELATES TO THAT'S ALL WE NEED.

IF YOU FEEL THE WORD COULD CAUSE EMBARRASSMENT OR YOU DON'T WANT TO DISCLOSE IT THAT'S PERFECTLY OK, INSTEAD YOU CAN ABBREVIATE IT OR CHOOSE A CODE WORD. LIKE 'A' 'B' 'C' OR ORANGE OR BANANNA.

THIS IS WHY EMDR IS NON VERBAL YOU NEVER NEED TO EXPLAIN OR DISCUSS OR ELABORATE ON WHAT THE MEANING OF THE WORD IS – IT'S CONFIDENTIAL TO YOU WE'RE NOT GOING TO TALK OR DISCUSS WHAT YOU WRITE OK?

SO TO BEGIN WE ARE JUST GOING TO START BY TAKING SOME DEEP BREATHS TO RELAX US A LITTLE, THIS HELPS WITH RECALLING ALL THOSE MEMORIES WE'RE LOOKNG FOR.

CLOSE YOUR EYES:

BREATHE IN FOR 4 FILLING YOUR LUNGS AND SHOULDERS

HOLD IT... HOLD IT...

BREATHE OUT SLOWLY FOR 8 EXHALE ALL THE AIR.

BREATHE IN FOR 4 FILLING YOUR LUNGS AND SHOULDERS.

HOLD IT... HOLD IT...

BREATHE OUT SLOWLY FOR 8 EXHALE ALL THE AIR.

BREATHE IN FOR 4 FILLING YOUR LUNGS AND SHOULDERS.

HOLD IT... HOLD IT... HOLD IT...

BREATHE OUT SLOWLY FOR 8 EXHALE ALL THE AIR.

OPEN YOUR EYES FEELING SO MUCH MORE RELAXED.

(Using a black or blue pen YOU draw a medium sized circle in the top left corner of the page)

SO THERE'S OUR FIRST CIRCLE.

IN A MINUTE YOU'RE GOING TO WRITE JUST ONE OR TWO WORDS IN THAT CIRCLE.

WRITE THE NAME OR USE A CODE WORD OF A TRAUAMTIC MEMORY, THOUGHT OR FEELING.

AS SOON AS YOU'VE WRITTEN IN THE CIRCLE DRAW ANOTHER CIRCLE THE SAME SIZE TO THE RIGHT OF THE FIRST CIRCLE.

FOCUS ON THE BLANK CIRCLE YOU'VE JUST DRAWN, BY DOING THIS YOU WON'T FOCUS ON WHAT YOU'VE JUST WRITTEN.

JUST WRITE ONE OR TWO WORDS IN THAT CIRCLE OF ANOTHER TRAUMATIC MEMORY, THOUGHT OR FEELING, JUST WRITE WHAT COMES INTO YOUR MIND.

DRAW ANOTHER CIRCLE AND WRITE WHAT COMES INTO YOUR MIND.

DRAW ANOTHER CIRCLE AND WRITE WHAT COMES INTO YOUR MIND.

(if the subject doesn't draw a circle simply ask them quietly to DRAW A CIRCLE and point to the place where the circle should be drawn, remind them to FOCUS ON THE BLANK CIRCLE they have just drawn)

(let them continue until they become stuck or have finished)

(if they are STUCK and they will say this or just not write anything)

IF YOU FEEL STUCK JUST CLOSE YOUR EYES:

BREATHE IN FILLING YOUR LUNGS AND SHOULDERS.

HOLD IT... HOLD IT...

BREATHE OUT SLOWLY EXHALE ALL THE AIR.

BREATHE IN FILLING YOUR LUNGS AND SHOULDERS.

HOLD IT... HOLD IT...

BREATHE OUT SLOWLY EXHALE ALL THE AIR.

BREATHE IN FILLING YOUR LUNGS AND SHOULDERS.

HOLD IT... HOLD IT... HOLD IT...

BREATHE OUT SLOWLY EXHALE ALL THE AIR.

WITH YOUR EYES CLOSED CONTINUE TO BREATHE NORMALY. IN A MOMENT I'M GOING TO ASK YOU TO OPEN YOUR EYES, AND WHEN I DO FOCUS SOFTLY ON THE CIRCLE YOU'VE JUST DRAWN AND WRITE WHAT COMES INTO YOUR MIND.

OPEN YOUR EYES AND WRITE WHAT COMES INTO YOUR MIND.

(the subject will start to write again and the process continues - if they become stuck again simply ask the subject to close their eyes and instruct them in the breathing exercise all over again)

(at some point the subject will just stop and they will categorically KNOW they have finished. It's a very different feeling and body language to someone who is 'stuck'. Once they have finished you can move onto the next step, but only after you've checked everything you need to cover is recorded in one of the circles drawn?)

AS YOU NOW LOOK OVER EVERYTHING THAT YOU'VE WRITTEN IS THERE ANYTHING YOU CAN REMEMBER THAT YOU'VE LEFT OUT, IS THERE ANYTHING ELSE YOU'D LIKE TO ADD OR WORK ON?

(That question will lead to two possible answers; NO or YES, and if it's a YES simply ask the subject to draw another circle and label that memory. Remember to ask the same question again! Don't assume there was only one memory left out)

(what we have covered here is an INDIRECT approach where the subject directs the therapy and brings forward what they are happy to work on, if you are concerned they haven't addressed the issues you are aware of change the approach to become DIRECTED by you)

IS THE ISSUE YOU MENTIONED ON HERE?

(again the subject will answer YES and probably show you - they may have described or labelled the memory in a different way to what you were expecting, but if NO, just ask them to draw a circle and label that memory)

(if they chose not to you must respect that decision and do not push the subject or they will simply not engage in the process. Perhaps come back to the circle when they feel more comfortable and move on to the next phase)

YOU'VE DONE REALLY WELL!

(move straight on avoid discussing what has been written)

NOW WE NEED TO GRADE THEM, FOR THIS WE USE A RED PEN.

NOW GRADE THE MEMORIES BY WRITING A NUMBER IN EACH CIRCLE FROM 0 – 10. FEEL THE NUMBER DON'T THINK IT, YOUR MIND WILL INTUITIVLEY KNOW WHAT THE NUMBER IS. 0 IS THE LOWEST AND 10 IS THE HIGHEST.

THIS NUMBER REPRESENTS HOW 'BOTHERED' YOU ARE BY WHAT'S WRITTEN IN THE CIRCLE, OR HOW PAINFUL IT FEELS, OR HOW DISTRESSING THE MEMORY IS WHEN YOU THINK ABOUT IT.

WRITE THE NUMBER IN EACH CIRCLE IN RED, THEN MOVE STRAIGHT ONTO THE NEXT CIRCLE AND JUST KEEP GOING THERES NO NEED TO DWELL, JUST WRITE THE NUMBER THAT FIRST COMES INTO YOUR MIND.

(as they write add up the numbers, to give you the total number)

(once you have the total you can refer them back to the ANXIETY GRAPH you've drawn for them and show them where they now sit on that chart)

(it's at this stage for the first time they actually realise why they feel the way they feel, because they can see it on the graph – point it out on the graph)

SO THIS IS WHY YOU FEEL THE WAY YOU DO BECAUSE OF THE ACCUMULATIVE EFFECT OF THE TRAUMAS YOUVE GONE THROUGH WHICH ADDS UP TO .... (say the total number) WHICH RELATES TO HOW STRESSED OR ANXIOUS YOU FEEL.

A SCORE BETWEEN 25-50 MEANS YOU WILL FEEL STRESS.

A SCORE BETWEEN 50-75 MEANS YOU WILL BE EXPERIENCING ANXIETY IN YOUR DAILY LIFE AND YOUR BEHAVIOUR WILL START TO CHANGE AS YOUR MIND STARTS TO DISTRACT ITSELF FROM THE ANXIETY IT'S FEELING.

AND OVER 75 IS WHERE WE PERHAPS START TO SEE REAL PHYSICAL CHANGES IN THE BODY.

NOW YOU'VE SEEN THAT PROBABLY FOR THE FIRST TIME EVER, DOES THAT MAKE SENSE AS TO WHY YOU'RE FEELING THE WAY YOU ARE?

SO NOW WE'RE GOING TO WORK OUT WHICH MEMORIES WE ACTUALLY NEED TO WORK ON AND WHICH ONES WE CAN CROSS OFF.

WE CAN NOW DELETE ANY MEMORY GRADED 4 OR LOWER, ONLY IF YOU FEEL IT'S OK TO REMOVE IT.

(go through the memory map and find any circle graded 4 or under)

(each memory graded a 5 is on the border line, some memories can be deleted, perhaps others should stay and be worked on, it's the subject's choice)

HERE'S A .... (say the red number in the circle) IF YOU FEEL IT SHOULD STAY THEN JUST LET ME KNOW AND WE CAN LEAVE IT THERE TO WORK ON.

ONCE THE HIGHER GRADED MEMORIES HAVE BEEN REPROCESSED YOUR MIND WILL USUALLY START TO THEN PROCESS THESE LOWER GRADE TRAUMAS ON THEIR OWN.

SO YOU SEE WE DON'T NEED TO TREAT EVERY MEMORY YOU'VE EVER HAD.

(but before you do always ask permission before crossing any one out – find the memories 4 and under and ask if you can delete them and put a line through each one)

IS IT OK to cross out THIS ONE?

(if they are unsure KEEP the circle)

AND THIS ONE?

(if there are no memories 5 or under then JUMP TO MOVING ON*)

WELL DONE THAT'S A GREAT START!

BY DELETING THESE WE'VE NOW ALREADY REDUCED THE NUMBER OF MEMORIES WE NEED TO TREAT SPEEDING UP YOUR TREATMENT.

*MOVING ON – WE'RE NOW GOING TO SPEED UP THE PROCESS SAFELY AGAIN BY GROUPING THE REMAINING MEMORIES WHERE POSSIBLE.

ARE ANY OF THESE MEMORIES CONNECTED, HAVE ANY OF THE MEMORIES HERE HAPPENED AT THE SAME TIME, IF SO CAN THEY BE GROUPED?

POINT OUT THE ONES THAT ARE GROUPED AND I'LL DRAW A LINE CONNECTNG THEM, THERE'S NO NEED TO EXPLAIN WHY.

(now draw a line between each circle joining them together, there maybe 3-10 circles grouped, just draw a line between each one, if lines start to cross draw two very small straight lines like a bridge or brackets recording the direction of flow)

GREAT NOW WE'VE GROUPED ALL THOSE WE CAN WORK ON THEM AS A GROUP AT THE SAME TIME, SO NOW WE HAVE....... (add up the number of groups and single memories on the paper) AREAS OF TRAUMA TO TREAT RATHER THAN........ (say the total starting number before deletion and grouping).

YOU CAN SEE HOW GROUPING MEMORIES SPEEDS UP THE TREATMENT PROCESS.

WE'RE NOW GOING TO MOVE ONTO THE ACTUAL EMDR.

(go to **STEP 2- 'FIND'** script for adults)

So now we know how to carry out the standard MEMORY MAPPING process and what to say exactly, we are now going to look at how and why we adapt this for older and younger children.

When you come to actually treating adults or children, the script we've just covered is duplicated again at the rear of the book for ease of reference. You will find this script has been joined together with the phase 2, 3, and 4 scripts to make one full complete script, so you won't need to flick through the book to find each relevant section, for ease of use and to keep things simple. The scripts and learning have also been repeated as it is widely recognised repetition is a good way of learning to take all this new information in.

CHAPTER 9

Step 1 – 'FIND' for Older Children

Some quite older children may able to use the adult version of the MEMORY MAPPING process and that's great. If however you or they feel they would benefit from using more playful ways of mapping memories then you can use this unique process below. It's important to understand this process is exactly the same as for the adults, the outcome is the same, as is the aim and objective, it's how we go about explaining what we are doing and how it's going to work that differs. For this we have brought to real life the magic of spells, wands and wizards to carry out the process of Memory Mapping!

For older children the breathing technique to relax the mind is exactly the same. Begin with this.

It is helpful to then explain what we are trying to achieve, drawing the ANXIETY GRAPH may not be of any benefit, but if treating quite older children, educating them about how anxiety builds from a young age will be life changing for them, so if you feel it's age appropriate then use this or both systems together.

How to explain to a child what Anxiety is?

One way we have found very helpful that children respond well to is to tell one of the many stories that exist in many cultures, TV and film of a Dark Wizard who tries to enter children's minds with his dark magic, and when he does he can make them do things they wouldn't do normally which changes their behaviour. A perfect description of Anxiety!

We will be able to teach our children a spell called PROTECTO to keep the Dark Wizard out of their heads and we are going to teach you how you can use this later on in this book to teach children in the real world how to use magical spells to keep out unhelpful thoughts or anxiety. In real life we call this MINDFULNESS, in EASY EMDR here it's called MIND MAGIC!

Magic is creative way for children to visualise the process of finding memories, we have found it's easy to understand, learn and put into practice. We need to follow the same system as adults to carry out the MEMORY MAPPING but we are going to use real magic from the world of wizards!

The Memory Extraction Spell

Let's face it kids can get easily bored! If we use the traditional EMDR protocol with them they will very quickly lose interest and will not focus or engage with the process, and the EMDR will not work! This is one of the biggest challenges facing EMDR Therapists working with children. But now we have a solution that's fun and engaging!

First we need to set up the role play to bring the magic to life! I use a generic toy wand bought from a shop for wizards but any wand will do or even a stick, the same sheet of A4 paper and clip board, blue/black and red pens, and a magical 'Memory Flask', jar or bottle to hold the extracted memories in, very importantly it must not have a label on it and it must be ROUND!

The actual Memory Flask I use is made of vintage cut glass with an ornate silver top – it really helps to set the scene and recreate the magic that will make the process fun, thereby engaging and trusting for children – find objects that make it believable!

Flasks have been used throughout history in every culture to hold magic, like genies, potions, spells and memories. Here memories can be extracted by using a wand from the side of the head and the chosen memory then placed inside the bottle and labelled accordingly – the spell we use is EXTRACTO!

To be able to view the memory we use an age old magical device the 'Crystal Ball' which we use to place the memory into, and there it swirls around and the child can then 'look into' or focus on the Crystal Ball or magical circle, able to view the chosen memory. Some children may prefer to use the image of a witches' cauldron, there are many other magical devices that can be used as featured in lots of children's wizarding movies and TV programs, like magic wells with broomsticks, and magical plates or mirrors. I remember a lucky magic well from my own childhood at the bottom of my grandmas' garden!

This is the equipment I use; a wand, memory flask and a crystal ball!

We use exactly the same Adult Memory Mapping process except we explain it using our magical objects, and spells to engage the child's mind fully.

So now you know how to carry out our Memory Mapping for adults, now we are going to adapt this for older children who understand magic or who have seen any of the many Wizarding movies. Even if they haven't I've included an image here (with sincere thanks to Lyla-Rose Dunkley our child model), to help you explain in a fun magical way how a child can pull out and label memories from their minds.

Using the Wand

It is important to explain the process to them in a playful way, so in order for them to feel better about .... (insert the problem they are facing) you're going to help them, by removing the sad or upsetting memory from their head and giving them the choice to magic it away, and when it goes they will feel so much better.

After explaining the magic to the child and showing them the illustrations of the wand process (which you can find in Chapter 16), YOU place the wand at the child's temple and ask them to think of the memory that they would like to remove from their mind using the spell EXTRACTO.

Older children will understand the physical concept that parts of them can be removed or taken away and so will be able to allow the memory to be extracted. Once they have thought of the memory explain to the child you are now going to pull the memory out by using the wand and ask them to imagine it appearing as seen in the picture like a bright light.

Describe the memory being pulled out, describe the light appearing, and now comment on how you can see it and inform the child they can see it too! The child will inevitably agree. If they do they are now 'engaged' in the process.

If they choose not to see the memory they are not engaged in the process and you should then ask the child why they cannot see the memory? It is always important to go back and explain to them in order for them to feel better you are going to help them by removing the memory from their mind and giving the child the choice to 'pull it out' with the wand using EXTRACTO.

Ask them if they are now ready to pull out the memory from their mind, and once they agree you can continue with placing the wand lightly against the child's temple.

Pull the memory out slowly and comment on how you can both now see this now attached to the wand like a bright light.

Bottling and Labelling Memories

Make sure you have your Memory Flask to hand, or the empty jar or bottle with a lid ensuring there is NO label on the flask.

Describe the object as a magical device that will safely store the memory where the child can still see it, ensure the flask is always seen by the child and they do not look away.

Keep their focus on the memory be describing playfully how you are now putting the tip of the wand into the memory flask and shaking the memory off so it falls into the flask, and then describe how you can see it swirling around and place the lid on the flask or your finger.

Straight away point out acting surprised OH NO there's NO label! Ask out loud: How do we know what this memory is? You can exclaim "I know!" Excitedly explain to the child, what should we call it? Ask the child to give the memory a label, a description, ask them for just one or two words to describe what they would like to call it?

The child will then give you a name that is the WORD. Now take the flask with the memory called ...... and use the name they've given you. Now POUR the memory into the crystal ball, or instead just draw a circle on your A4 paper, and explain the circle represents a crystal ball etc. Now write the name of the memory in that circle as if using the ADULT protocol. So now you have completed one circle!

You can now draw another circle on the paper exactly the same as before. Write the label or the name of the memory in the circle and praise the child.

Explain now you are going to pull out another sad or upsetting memory with the wand. Take the top off the flask and turn the flask to face the child so they can see into the flask or bottle, show them the ROUND circle shape of the top of the flask is what you've drawn on the paper, so the round circles on the paper now represent the top and opening of each flask – this bypasses you pouring the memory into the circle, teaching the child in stages, to then just write the memories straight into the circle bypassing the flask!

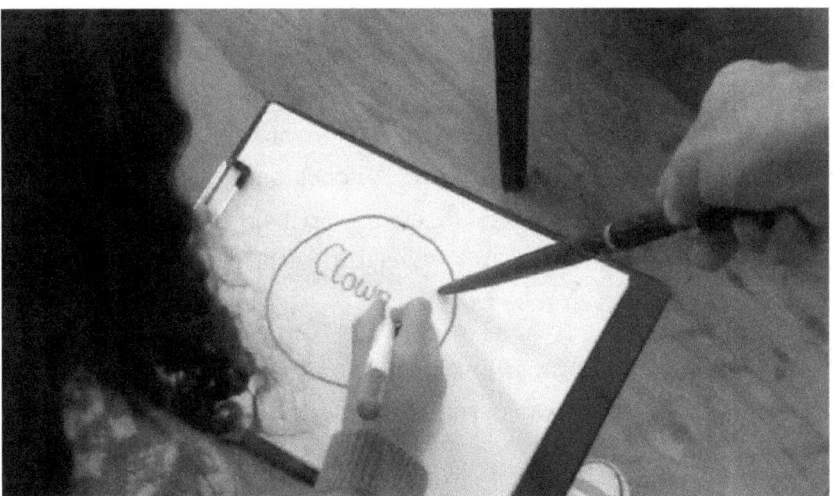

Now take the wand again and this time explain you are going to take the memory and put into directly into the top of the flask you've drawn, and pull out another memory and move the wand so the tip is in the middle of the circle.

Ask the child to name the memory and write the word in the circle. You now have the second memory recorded but you've speeded up the process by cutting out the use of the flask.

You can put the flask to one side now (unless the child likes using it) as we are just going to use the circles. For the third memory put the wand away, instead take the blue/black pen, and explain to the child they can use this as if it was a wand! Give the pen to the child, ask THEM to draw the next circle or flask for the next memory.

Ask them to put the bottom end of the pen (not the point) close to the temple and ask them to use this as if it was a wand, instruct them to now use the pen to pull out the next memory, just like the wand, direct them to place the memory into the next circle, just like the flask, and straight away ask them to write in the circle the name or label for this memory.

Now not only have you successfully recorded 3 memories which are effectively the areas of trauma that you will go on to target with the EASY EMDR treatment, but you've just taught your child in a fun and playful way, the adult protocol version of Memory Mapping by bringing into real life the magic of Witches and Wizards! They can now just write their troubles in circles on paper during the home therapy, or even afterward in a special magical diary! You can then use this special diary at the next session!

Now you've achieved this for three memories just keep going until the child is either stuck or finished.

If the child is stuck simply follow the same adult protocol for being 'stuck' as above. Again the child will know when they are finished. Once you have all the circles completed you will now be able to move onto the actual EASY EMDR, and this is where you will use the Magic Circle as a representation of the crystal ball or mirror etc.

What we have covered here is an INDIRECT approach where the child directs the therapy and brings forward what they are happy to work on, this is always the best approach to start.

However if you are working with a family member and you know some of the child's history and you are concerned they haven't addressed the issues you discussed, then you can change the approach to become DIRECTED.

All this means is you now direct the therapy and to do this you can simply ask them directly "Is the issue (you can name the subject matter) we discussed recorded here" Again the subject may answer YES and probably show you (they may have described or labelled the memory in a different way to what you were expecting – recall the CHERRY TREE example), or NO, again ask them to draw a circle and label that memory.

If they chose not to you must respect that decision and do not push the subject or they will simply not engage in the process. Perhaps come back to the therapy when they feel more comfortable.

Grading the Memories

This process is exactly the same as we've already learnt for the ADULTS, but with a little less explanation as children can learn the therapy techniques that underpin EASY EMDR for perhaps later in life. You can use this book to teach them as they grow older so they can even use it with their children!

Again in order to grade the memories once all the circles have been drawn we use a RED pen to help create stand out from all the written detail. For this I use the 'Bothered O Meter' which you can redraw like this ad use your pen as the arrow, or make an arrow and attach it to a cardboard image:

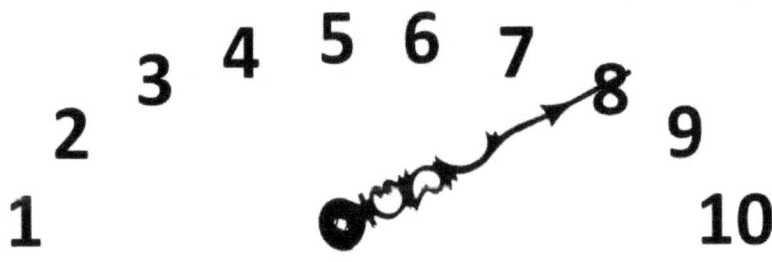

Ask the child to GRADE the memories by writing a number in each circle from 0 – 10. Explain to the child to FEEL the number not THINK of it they will be able to do this if you describe it as the "first number that comes into their head". Explain to the child 0 is low and 10 is high. Explain to the subject this number represents how 'bothered' they are by the memory in the circle, there's no need to mention how painful it feels, or how distressing the memory is – let's save that for the adults!

This should be a very easy process, one which I have experienced full and complete success with every child treated within clinic.

At the end of the process add up the numbers. They will give you a total of perhaps 34, or 56, or 79 or 98 up to 100 is very common. Children will rarely go over 100 as they haven't lived long enough to experience such a high total accumulation of traumas, however it is possible as one child I have treated recorded over 800 SUD's.

Once you have the total you can refer back to the ANXIETY GRAPH ONLY IF YOU ARE USING IT and show them where they are on that chart. It's at this stage that often a moment of euphoria happens as the child for the first time actually realises why they feel the way they feel, because they can see it on the graph.

So it's important to explain to them, this is why they feel the way they do because of the accumulative effect of all the historical traumas they've gone through, add up to a number which relates to how worried they may feel.

Remind them, a total score between 0-25 means they will not feel stressed, a score between 25-50 means they will feel stress, a score between 50-75 means they will be experiencing anxiety in their daily lives and their behaviours will start to change as the mind starts to distract it from the anxiety its feeling, and over 75 means they are suffering from acute anxiety and may even feel the need to self-harm or have suicidal thoughts.

Don't be afraid about using these explanations with older children, including mentioning suicide if it is age appropriate, as educating older children about anxiety will teach them when to ask for help, before they self-harm, have thoughts of suicide or their behaviours change irreversibly and it becomes too late to intervene.

As I mentioned before this, education is vital in the early intervention of mental health and if you can teach your child to recognise and ask for help then you will be breaking the negative harmful cycle of child and even adult mental health issues!

Deleting low grade Memories

We again now need to DELETE any memory graded 4 or lower by crossing them out with a RED line through the circle. Ask if it's OK to cross out any memory graded lower than a 5! As a 5 is on the border line some memories can be deleted, perhaps others should stay and be worked on, and it's the child's choice. If they are unsure KEEP the circle. So again we can safely perhaps delete even more speeding up the process even more!

Grouping Memories

We are now going to speed up the process safely again by grouping memories where possible. Ask the child if any of the memories happened at the same time, can they be grouped? Use those exact words. Here's the example used earlier which you can use again with some different words:

MEMORIES/LABELS IN CIRCLES:

1. CHERRY TREE
2. BREAKING LEGS
3. PAIN WALKING
4. BYCYCLE ACCIDENT
5. PETS DEATH

Now the subject says the first three are all connected, when they fell out of the CHERRY TREE they BROKE THEIR LEGS which went on to cause PAIN WALKING, so they are all CONNECTED and can be GROUPED by drawing a red line again. The 4th and 5th are separate, they happened later in the child's life you are told, so do NOT link these with a line.

The MEMORY MAP GROUPS will now look like this:

1. CHERRY TREE, BREAKING LEGS, PAIN WALKING
2. BYCYCLE ACCIDENT
3. PET'S DEATH

You can refer back to the illustrations in the previous Adult chapter if needed. When grouping you may find there are 5-10 circles grouped, just draw a line between each one. You may find that lines start to cross with multiple trauma MEMORY MAPS.

If they do simply draw two very small straight lines like brackets or map bridge symbol to record the direction of flow of lines that cross, as we have done before.

What if a child becomes distressed during Memory Mapping?

During the MEMORY MAPPING process it is possible the child may become distressed in that they may become sad, feel anxious or even cry.

This can seem frightening to anyone but it is important you remain focused and continue to guide the subject to draw the next circle etc. Often just this one action alone is enough to allow the subject to regain composure and move on and carry on.

Remember the Firework story? Perhaps you could chose to explain this to the child before starting the process. Here's a quick reminder;

"It's like a Firework going off! Sometimes they just sparkle with a little bang, sometimes they go off with a big bang! But soon as they do they ALL start to fizzle out and disappear and once a Firework has been lit and has gone off it can never be re-lit again – it's finished! It's Gone!".

But unlike real fireworks they are only memories they are thinking of not actually the real event so it cannot harm them even if they feel a little scared.

This is how EMDR works with even the most distressing of memories. The EYE MOVEMENT fizzles out or DESENSITISES the subject to the memory and then the mind REPROCESSES the memory so it doesn't come back! It's a simplistic, yet easy and very straight forward way of explaining what has always been a very complex treatment – until now we hope!

There can be very rare cases where a subject will not be able to carry on and may be overcome with emotion. When drawing the graph (if using) it will already become apparent very early on if the child is likely to experience what may appear to be uncontrollable emotion, as the child will already show signs of being very emotional.

In this instance, if you are aware this may happen it is important to distract the child from what they are feeling and we do this by simply taking them to a SAFE PLACE in their mind.

If the child shows signs of heightened emotion from the outset then it would always be best to set this up before starting any of the MEMORY MAPPING.

To set up a SAFE PLACE ask the child to first identify and name to you a place they consider to be safe; their home, bedroom, holiday, beach. It doesn't have to be safe to us, it is where they feel they can safely go to in their mind where no harm can come to them, a place where they are in control.

Once they have named this place ask them to close their eyes and imagine being there. You can help them by asking them to describe the location, room, temperature, colours, what they can see, but importantly how they feel. Once you know they feel safe you can explain to them they can go back to this place whenever YOU instruct them too and they will be safe.

You can test this by asking the subject to describe what they were doing yesterday and after a little while ask them firmly to CLOSE THEIR EYES AND GO TO YOUR SAFE PLACE NOW! Once they are there ask them to describe it again and how they feel, it will be the same as before. The child now knows they can proceed safely.

If during the MEMORY MAPPING process they become distressed enough that they cannot continue you MUST take control of the situation and immediately instruct them firmly to CLOSE THEIR EYES AND GO TO YOUR SAFE PLACE NOW!

Once they are there ask them to describe it again and how they feel, it will be the same as before. The child will begin to calm. Now use the 4 IN 8 OUT breathing technique you have already learnt and practiced. This will reduce the anxiety further, you can then stop & revisit this later or carry on.

If the subject chooses to continue with the process which is advisable, start on a new blank circle. Remember you can use this technique in the highly unlikely event your subject becomes overly distressed at any point during the EASY EMDR session. Feeling some emotional distress is a necessary part of this treatment, do not shy away from it but stick to the process, it will work and the emotional sensitivity will reduce.

I have had a number of cases where the subject could have given up, but we persisted and the EMDR worked as it should to reduce the trauma. I will explain how we do this later on in the following chapters.

It is important to only intervene where absolutely necessary, as if you do so every time the child shows a little emotion you will never be able to target the actual trauma, and when we come on to do this it is very common that there is always some degree of distress, as we are recalling sad or upsetting memories not happy ones. Again there's lots more on this later.

No matter what you do they are already aware of the memories so you cannot make anything worse or bring up feelings that were hidden or repressed as they are already in the child's conscious memory. To do this again you would need to use Clinical Hypnotherapy, which is why this book does NOT advocate or explain the use of Regression as this kind of therapy should only be carried out by trained and experienced therapists.

So now we know how in detail to carry out the MEMORY MAPPING for Older Children with or without MIND MAGIC, we can now go on to practice this step. I've written out the exact wording to use for the entire phase of this step of the treatment – this is what we call a 'script'.

Once you become proficient enough in its contents you can do away with it, it's just a guide to get you going. It's a synopsis of everything we've already covered before. I've put together the entire script and illustrations for 'Older Children' at Chapter 16 for quick and easy reference titled "How to conduct a Session – for Older Children".

MEMORY MAPPING SCRIPT - OLDER CHILDREN

Some quite older children may able to use the adult version of the MEMORY MAPPING process and that's great – refer to that.

If however you or they feel they would benefit from using more playful ways of mapping memories then you can use this script instead:

It's important to understand this process is exactly the same as for the adults, the outcome is the same, as is the aim and objective, but for this we have instead brought to life the magic of spells!

So before we start anything let's help the child create that safe space. Remember if your child shows signs of heightened emotion from the outset then it would always be best to set this up before starting any of the MEMORY MAPPING.

(explain the fireworks story)

SOMETIMES WHEN WE FIX THE SAD MEMORIES IN OUR HEAD IT CAN BE LIKE A FIREWORK GOING OFF!

SOMETIMES THEY JUST SPARKLE WITH A LITTLE BANG, SOMETIMES THEY GO OFF WITH A BIG BANG! BUT SOON AS THEY DO THEY ALL START TO FIZZLE OUT AND DISAPPEAR.

ONCE A FIREWORK HAS BEEN LIT AND HAS GONE OFF IT CAN NEVER BE RE-LIT AGAIN CAN IT? IT'S FINISHED! IT'S GONE!

SO IF WE FIND ONES WITH BIG BANGS AND WE GET A BIT SCARED DON'T WORRY THEY'RE NOT ACTUALY REAL.

AND WE CAN ALWAYS GO TO A SAFE NICE PLACE – I'LL SHOW YOU HOW:

CAN YOU THINK OF A SAFE NICE PLACE RIGHT NOW? WHERE WOULD YOU LIKE TO GO TO FEEL SAFE? HOW ABOUT YOUR HOME, BEDROOM, ON HOLIDAY OR NICE BEACH!

(a child's home or bedroom may not be safe for a child so expect anything to come up, if so ask them to create a magical space in their mind. Once they've named this place ask them to close their eyes)

THAT'S A NICE PLACE, NOW CLOSE YOUR EYES AND IMAGINE BEING THERE. CAN YOU TELL ME ABOUT WHERE YOU ARE WHAT COLOURS AND THINGS CAN YOU SEE - HOW DO YOU FEEL?

(once you know they feel safe go on to explain)

NOW YOU CAN GO BACK TO THIS PLACE WHENEVER I ASK YOU TO AND YOU WILL BE SAFE, LETS TRY IT NOW.

WHAT DID YOU DO YESTERDAY?

(let them talk and after a little while ask them firmly)

CLOSE YOUR EYES AND GO TO YOUR SAFE PLACE NOW! CAN YOU DESCRIBE IT AGAIN TO ME - AND HOW DO YOU NOW FEEL?

(your subject will begin to calm. Now use the 4 IN 8 OUT breathing technique you have already learnt and practised. This will reduce the anxiety)

(remember: If during the MEMORY MAPPING process they become distressed enough that they cannot continue you MUST take control of the situation and instruct them firmly to listen to your voice)

(it is important to only intervene where absolutely necessary)

(it is helpful to first explain to the older child what we are trying to achieve, drawing the Anxiety Graph will probably be of no benefit, but if treating older children then educating them about how anxiety builds from a young age will be life changing for them, so if you feel its age appropriate then DO use this graph or both systems together)

(do that now if appropriate)

TO HELP YOU RESOLVE THE FEELINGS AND THOUGHTS AND ANXIETY YOU'VE BEEN HAVING I'M JUST GOING TO TALK YOU THROUGH THIS SIMPLE GRAPH SO WE UNDERSTAND WHY YOU'VE BEEN FEELING THE WAY DO.

THIS GRAPH IS THEN GOING TO HELP US IDENTIFY THE CAUSES AND THAT'S WHAT WE ARE THEN GOING TO USE THE EASY EMDR ON, TO RESOLVE THOSE FEELINGS & MEMORIES.

(Explain and talk through the anxiety graph – a copy of which can be found at Chapter 16.)

(but if this explanation is not age appropriate miss out the graph completely and perhaps use the explanation script below to teach a child what Anxiety is WITHOUT the graph)

THOSE FEELINGS AND MEMORIES CAN FEEL LIKE BEING UNDER A SPELL WHICH MAKES CHILDREN DO THINGS THEY WOULDN'T NORMALLY AND CHANGE THEIR BEHAVIOR.

AS WE KNOW THERE ARE GOOD SPELLS AND BAD SPELLS, THE BAD SPELLS MAKE US FEEL UNWELL, THE GOOD SPELLS HELP US GET WELL.

WHAT WE ARE GOING TO DO NOW IS USE THE GOOD SPELLS TO MAKE US FEEL SO MUCH BETTER.

NOW TO BE ABLE TO DO MAGIC WE NEED A WAND, HERE WE ARE! AND WE CAN USE A CRYSTAL BALL, SOME PAPER AND A PEN AND A MAGICAL 'MEMORY FLASK', TO CONTAIN THE MEMORIES IN.

(show the child all these items and let them explore them)

MEMORY FLASKS HAVE BEEN USED THROUGHOUT MAGICAL HISTORY IN EVERY CULTURE TO HOLD THINGS LIKE GENIES, POTIONS, SPELLS & MEMORIES.

WHAT WE ARE GOING TO DO IS USE THE MAGIC WAND TO FIND OUR SAD MEMORIES AND EXTRACT THEM WITH THE WAND FROM OUR HEAD AND PUT THE CHOSEN MEMORY INSIDE THE BOTTLE.

THEN WE ARE GOING TO GIVE THE MEMORY A NAME AND LABEL THE BOTTLE.

TO BE ABLE TO LOOK AT THE MEMORY WE USE AN OLD MAGICAL DEVICE A 'CRYSTAL BALL' WHICH IS LIKE A MAGIC CIRCLE, AND WE USE IT TO PLACE THE MEMORY INTO, AND THERE IT SWIRLS AROUND SO WE WILL BE ABLE TO SEE THE MEMORY!

AND THEN THAT'S IT DA DAH!! WE'VE FOUND THE MEMORY USING MAGIC!

LET'S HAVE A GO.

(you can show the child the illustrations of what you're about to do to make it easy to explain and understand in Chapter 16)

OK SO I TAKE HOLD OF THE WAND, AND PUT IT TO MY HEAD AND NOW I THINK OF THE SAD MEMORY.... HMMM THERE IT IS! NOW I SLOWLY PULL OUT THE MEMORY LIKE A BUBBLE AND AS IT STICKS TO THE END OF THE WAND LIKE A SPARKLY SPELL I POP IT INTO THE MEMORY FLASK!

(Describe the memory as a bright light being pulled out, describe the memory appearing and comment on how you can see it and inform the child they can see it too as you place it into the flask. The child will inevitably agree. They are now 'engaged' in the process)

OK NOW YOU TRY! BUT BEFORE THAT WE ARE GOING TO SAFELY ENTER A MAGICAL SPACE NICE AND CALM TOGETHER:

CLOSE YOUR EYES.

NOW BREATHE IN FILLING YOUR BODY UP WITH AIR.

HOLD IT... HOLD IT...

AND BREATHE OUT SLOWLY KEEP YOUR EYES CLOSED.

BREATHE IN AGAIN THAT'S RIGHT ALL THE WAY IN.

HOLD IT.... HOLD IT...

AND BREATHE OUT ALL THE AIR SLOWLY.

AND ONE MORE TIME BREATHE ALL THE WAY IN.

HOLD IT... HOLD IT... HOLD IT...

AND BREATHE OUT SLOWLY.

AND OPEN YOUR EYES FEELING NICE AND CALM.

NOW PLACE THE WAND ON THE SIDE OF YOUR HEAD THAT'S RIGHT AND THINK OF THE MEMORY THAT YOU WOULD LIKE TO REMOVE.

ONCE YOU'VE THOUGHT OF THE MEMORY YOU'RE NOW GOING TO PULL THE MEMORY OUT IN A BUBBLE BY USING THE WAND AND IMAGINE IT APPEARING AS THAT BRIGHT LIGHT (use the illustrations).

(if they chose not to see the bubble or light - that's why we give them two options, they are not engaged in the process)

(you should then ask the child why they cannot see the memory. It is important to go back and explain to them in order for them to feel better you are going to help them by removing the memory from their mind and giving the child the choice to let it go away by using the wand)

(once they agree continue again placing the wand at the child's temple)

OK SO NOW PULL THE MEMORY OUT THAT'S RIGHT THERE IT IS! THE MEMORY BUBBLE IS ATTACHED TO THE WAND.

(make sure you have your Memory Flask to hand, or the empty jar or bottle with a lid ensuring there is NO label on the flask)

NOW WE PUT THE MEMORY INTO THE MAGICAL FLASK THAT WILL SAFELY STORE THE MEMORY WHERE YOU CAN STILL SEE IT – THAT'S RIGHT IN IT GOES!

(ensure the flask is always seen by the child and they do not look away)

AND THERE IS YOUR MEMORY SWIRLING ALL AROUND.

(acting surprised and excited)

AH THERE IS NO LABEL! OH NO! HOW DO WE KNOW WHAT THIS MEMORY IS?

I KNOW! WE CAN GIVE THE MEMORY A LABEL, A NAME CAN'T WE.

OK HOW ABOUT YOU JUST GIVE ME ONE OR TWO WORDS TO DESCRIBE WHAT YOU'D LIKE TO CALL IT?

THAT'S REALLY GOOD WELL DONE! NOW YOU SEE THE TOP OF THE BOTTLE WHAT SHAPE IS IT?

(turn the bottle to face the child so they can see the round opening)

A CIRCLE THAT'S RIGHT, SO LET'S DRAW THE TOP OF THE BOTTLE ON THE PAPER - THERE WE GO A CIRCLE! THAT'S THE TOP OF OUR BOTTLE, AND WE CAN WRITE THE NAME .... ON THE BOTTLE.

(write the label the child has given you in the circle - you have now written in the circle as if using the ADULT protocol)

SO LETS DRAW ANOTHER CIRCLE, ANOTHER BOTTLE AND NOW LET'S FIND ANOTHER MEMORY AND PULL IT OUT AND PUT IT IN THE NEW BOTTLE JUST AS WE DID BEFORE.

(repeat the wand memory extraction process EXTRACTO again)

NOW TAKE THE WAND AGAIN AND THIS TIME YOU CAN TAKE THE MEMORY AND PUT INTO DIRECTLY INTO THE TOP OF THE FLASK WE'VE DRAWN, AND WRITE THE NAME OF THE MEMORY IN THAT CIRCLE – THAT'S RIGHT!

(you now have the second memory recorded but you've speeded up the process by cutting out the use of the flask. You can put this to one side now as we are just going to use the circles - you can buy a pen that looks like a wand if this helps)

NOW FOR THE THIRD MEMORY HOW ABOUT WE JUST USE THE PEN AS IF IT WAS A WAND! DRAW THE NEXT CIRCLE TO GET THE FLASK READY FOR THE NEXT MEMORY – THAT'S RIGHT.

NOW USE THE PEN AS YOUR WAND TO PULL OUT THE NEXT MEMORY, PLACE THE MEMORY INTO THE NEXT CIRCLE, AND WRITE IN THE CIRCLE THE NAME FOR THIS MEMORY.

(just keep going until the child is finished - if the child is stuck simply follow the same adult protocol for being 'stuck' by closing eyes and taking three breaths in and out)

(what we have covered here is an INDIRECT approach if you are concerned they haven't addressed the issues you discussed, then you can change the approach to become DIRECTED - simply ask them directly)

IS THE ISSUE OF .... (name the subject matter) WE DISCUSSED HERE ON THE PAPER SOMEWHERE?

(they may answer YES and show you but if it's a NO ask them to draw a circle and label that memory)

(if they chose not to, you must respect that decision and do not push the subject or they will simply not engage in the process, perhaps come back to the therapy when they feel more comfortable)

(once you have all the circles completed you will now be able to move onto grading the memories on the scale of BEING BOTHERED before you move onto the actual EMDR, where you will use the Magic Circles drawn as a representation of the Crystal Ball)

(in order to grade the memories use a RED pen)

WELL DONE SO NOW WE ARE GOING TO GRADE THE MEMORIES BY WRITING A NUMBER IN EACH CIRCLE FROM 0 – 10 – YOU WILL KNOW WHAT THE NUMBER IS, IT'S THE FIRST NUMBER THAT COMES INTO YOUR HEAD.

0 IS LOW AND 10 IS HIGH. THIS NUMBER REPRESENTS HOW 'BOTHERED' YOU ARE BY THE MEMORY IN THE CIRCLE, ITS VERY EASY JUST LOOK AT THAT MEMORY AND WRITE THE NUMBER IN THE CIRCLE THERE – WELL DONE! NOW KEEP GOING AND LETS GRADE THEM ALL.

(use the Bothered Scale illustration or draw it for them if needed)

(add up the numbers they will give you a total, once you have the total you can refer back to the Anxiety Graph to see where your child sits and if this is what you expected – explain this to them if using the adult script below)

SO THIS IS WHY YOU FEEL THE WAY YOU DO BECAUSE OF THE TOTAL EFFECT OF THE TRAUMAS YOU'VE GONE THROUGH WHICH ADDS UP TO .... (say the total number) WHICH RELATES TO HOW STRESSED OR ANXIOUS YOU FEEL.

A SCORE BETWEEN 25-50 MEANS YOU WILL FEEL STRESS.

A SCORE BETWEEN 50-75 MEANS YOU WILL BE EXPERIENCING ANXIETY DAILY AND EVEN YOUR BEHAVIOUR WILL START TO CHANGE AS YOUR MIND STARTS TO DISTRACT ITSELF FROM THE ANXIETY IT'S FEELING.

AND OVER 75 IS WHERE WE PERHAPS START TO SEE REAL PHYSICAL CHANGES IN THE BODY (use the following statement if only age appropriate) AND YOU MAY EVEN FEEL LIKE SELF HARMING OR FEEL SUICIDAL.

NOW YOU'VE SEEN THAT PROBABLY FOR THE FIRST TIME EVER, DOES THAT MAKE SENSE AS TO WHY YOU ARE FEELING THE WAY YOU ARE?

(if using the non-adult version of the anxiety graph start again from here)

SO NOW WE'RE GOING TO WORK OUT WHICH MEMORIES WE NEED TO USE OUR MAGIC ON TO MAKE THEM DISAPEAR AND WHICH ONES WE DON'T SO WE CAN CROSS THEM OFF.

WE CAN NOW DELETE ANY MEMORY GRADED 4 OR LOWER, ONLY IF YOU FEEL IT'S OK TO REMOVE IT.

(any memory graded a 4 is on the border line some memories can be deleted, perhaps others should stay and be worked on, it's the child's choice)

IF YOU FEEL IT SHOULD STAY THEN JUST LET ME KNOW AND WE CAN LEAVE IT TO USE OUR MAGIC SPELLS ON.

(find the memories 4 and under and ask if you can delete and if yes put a line through each one)

IS IT OK to cross out THIS ONE?

(if they are unsure KEEP the circle)

AND THIS ONE?

(if there are no memories 4 or under then just simply move on*)

WELL DONE THAT'S A GREAT START!

(there is no need to group children's memories as they will not write enough to warrant this part of the therapy)

WE'RE NOW GOING TO MOVE ONTO THE MAGIC SPELL USING OUR WAND TO FORGET ALL THESE MEMORIES – WELL DONE! YOU'VE DONE REALLY... REALLY WELL!

(praise the child and go to Step 2 'FEEL' script for Older Children)

When you come to actually treating older children, the script we've just covered is duplicated again at the rear of the book for ease of reference with simple illustrations. You will find this script would have been joined with the Step 2, 3, and 4 scripts to make one full complete script, so you won't need to flick through the book to find each relevant section, for ease of use and to keep things simple.

The scripts have also been repeated as it is widely recognised that repetition is a good way of learning and will help you to take all this new and exciting important information in.

You will be able to read from this script in one go from start to finish for each group, Adults, Older Children and Younger Children, as opposed to hear where it's been broken down by each of the four steps.

So now we know how to carry out the MIND MAGIC MEMORY MAPPING process for Older Children we are now going to look at how and why and how we adapt this for the Younger Children.

Chapter 10

Step 1 – 'FIND' for Younger Children

Now we're going to look at how to work with younger children using a different age appropriate MEMORY MAPPPING method. By younger children we mean children of an age that would feel more comfortable playing with finger puppets and drawing, painting or modelling, so this could be used for children who are biologically older too so it's important to note that therefore even some older children may find some of this approach very beneficial.

How do you tell which system to use? Just try each one if you're unsure, you can't do any harm! You can mix or swop out elements from the two systems.

We have to remember that we are looking for memories that are traumatic, in adults and older children the subject will be able to have at least some comprehension of trauma in that when they think of the memory it causes them distress or how much they are 'bothered' by it. For younger children the concept of distress and trauma may be blurred and may often require more time and patience for the child to identify with what the memory is, and that the child can 'let go' safely and that its helpful to let the memory go.

As an example a child who has been abused or sexualised at a young age may not understand that this was wrong or traumatic. It's probable the child will have learnt this as normal behaviour or may identify with the memory as a game. Therefore the child may feel that there's nothing wrong with them, and therefore they will not feel any anxiety and therefore the EMDR simply won't work, because there is nothing for it to work on. However if they do feel anything, or their behaviour is changing in that they are displaying sexualised behaviour, or they are becoming very angry and aggressive then we can target these 'feelings' or 'behaviours' instead.

In some cases the child may not understand what happened is 'traumatic' and therefore doesn't cause them distress but their behaviour is changing, what would we do in this instance? We can try to talk to the child and ask them how they feel about the issue, this is a DIRECT approach.

Or we can ask them how do they feel and not mention the issue, and allow the child the space to come up with their own 'issues' and hope the subject is one of them, this is an INDIRECT approach. We've discussed these approaches before.

It may therefore seem that the Memory Mapping process for younger children is more complex, that is somewhat true, it does take a different approach that requires more time, but it is not necessarily more complex, in fact it can often be very simple, either way be prepared not to rush this process when working with younger children.

Overall the treatment of younger children is however balanced out with the majority of time being spent at the start rather than the end of the treatment. It's the other way around for older children and adults, it's easier to identify traumatic memories and map them and because there are probably more it will take longer to treat them when we come onto the actual EMDR stage.

But when working with younger children it is usual that we can only work on one memory at a time, so we don't really need to concern ourselves with producing a detailed MEMORY MAP, so we can make the process simpler and easier for the young child and yourself.

The process in its simplest form is this:

1. Identify one memory
2. Carry out EMDR to desensitise/reprocess that one memory only.
3. On another occasion (at least 48 hours later – I'll explain why later on) you can work on another memory and so on and so on.

So to begin we now need to first identify one memory.

The easiest way to try first of all is to be DIRECTIVE – just ask the young child "Do you remember when ……." If they can remember then you have achieved the first step. That's it! You will then be able to move straight onto Step 2 'FEEL' which we will cover in a later chapter.

If they cannot remember or do not understand how to verbalise the trauma or they don't see it as a trauma then they will not trigger anxiety and if they do not trigger anxiety then the EMDR may not work when we move onto Step 2 'FEEL'.

If a child cannot 'FIND the memory in Step 1 as being traumatic or is unable to verbalise the memory or the event, we have a very useful standardised and recognised psychotherapy we can use at home – and this is THERA PLAY a combination of Art and Therapy!

ART THERAPY and PLAY can be DIRECTIVE or INDIRECTIVE. In its simplest form, rather than ask a child "Do they remember when.." or "How do you feel about …" we ask them to either draw, paint, model or create a unique piece of art with paper, crayons, pencils, pens, glue, glitter, string etc. – this is what can also be called THERAPLAY.

Again it is seen as a specialised subject for therapists but it can be used by families to treat emerging mental health issues as an early intervention at no cost. Alternatively you can always wait until the child is older and use the previous systems for older children but then you must be prepared to allow the child's behaviours to change over the years as the trauma becomes stored in the child's mind, affecting their relationships at home, their school, and their perception of themselves and their life around them as they grow up.

If you can intervene in the early years at the very least you will be teaching your younger child to engage and understand therapy ready for later on in their life, and at the very best you will be able to quickly and easily heal your child's mind and allow them to enjoy their childhood as a child should, being free from the stress, anxiety and worry that accompanies trauma.

In order to achieve this change it is very important that the child trusts the adult. When working with an unknown therapist initially this will be the goal to establish trust, so they child will feel safe to open up and tell or show the therapist their feelings and memories. This often takes place in a therapy setting in a strange unfamiliar room, which can also effect the time it takes to establish a trust relationship with working with a professional therapist.

This is where you as a parent, guardian or trusted family member have a definite significant advantage over professional therapists working in clinical settings, if you're lucky enough to be able to even access one of these. For some parents they cannot access a charity nearby or afford such professional help privately, in some countries this professional help does not even physically exist.

There are a small number of incredible charities that exist to support younger children and families and it is always advised where absolutely possible to seek out their professional help.

But often even these charities at present have no or little access to EMDR to actually treat the child after they have successfully used Theraplay or any other forms of therapy to identify and resolve trauma, and even then most EMDR therapists have little or no experience of how to treat younger children and therefore lack the confidence to even try. EMDR training for younger children at this time is not readily accessible or widely accessible.

So as a parent you can now take control of your children's mental health issues and you can learn how to help them instead. EASY EMDR for younger children bridges this gap and it does this well. The child will already trust you, and you are therefore already past the most challenging stage of the process – building trust. You can draw upon this established trust to help the child feel free and open to explore how they feel. Traditionally in therapy we look at this model as being a triangle. Unknowingly we've already used this triangular model when MEMORY MAPPING adult or older child memories.

The Triangle of Trust

The **'Triangle of Trust'** as we call it is made up here of the CHILD, the ADULT (or Therapist) and the OBJECT (the memory). The object is the CIRCLE as we've drawn before, but if the younger child cannot identify with this system then the OBJECT is the ART; the DRAWING, MODEL, PAINTING, COLLAGE etc.

This triangle is central to the EASY EMDR process, without it the subject will not engage in the process and the EMDR will not work.

Creating the Object

Invite the child to join you to do some Drawing, Painting, Modelling, Collage etc. Give them a choice of 'which ONE to choose'! That way you are ensuring they will not be given a reason to say NO, find what they like would like to do and you will thereby ensure their minds are already saying YES, by choosing their preferred art therapy.

So the OBJECT represents the memory we are looking to target with the EASY EMDR. All we have to do is give the younger child the creative space to draw, paint, model, build etc. and the art materials to do so.

Start by explaining to the child together you are now going to have play and create some art, use the words you would normally use to do this, at a time when you would normally do this, so the process is familiar and the younger child is at ease and 'trusting' from the outset, build this into a child's routine. Use the opportunity a familiar routine presents. If you don't have a routine based around art, you can start to create one just to have some fun, without the need to jump in right at the start with Theraplay.

When you are both ready, ask the younger child what they would like to use, what medium they prefer, and the process has begun positively. Then simply allow the child to create! Now here is where you decide which process you are going to employ. You can be INDIRECTIVE and just see what they create, or you can be DIRECTIVE and ask them to create art specifically about the issue you know needs work on, or there's another more effective option!

You can begin with an INDIRECTIVE approach and then if the younger child allows you, you can perhaps 'steer' the creative process a certain way, by you adding to the art work, introducing the subject matter you feel you need to work on, so you are now introducing 'direction' which is what the DIRECTIVE approach is ultimately all about! Don't take over, just steer and guide the process gently.

As the art unfolds you can ask 'open' engaging questions like: "That looks interesting, what's that? who's that? etc."

Avoid saying words like "that looks NICE or BEAUTIFUL" as the art may NOT represent to the child something positive, and by using these words you will either confuse or create distrust. It's always far better to keep questions and comments NEUTRAL.

If the child does begin to tell you what the art is and they are explaining or expressing the distressing memory, you've achieved your aim there and then and you should seize the moment and move straight onto Step 2 of EASY EMDR - 'FEEL'.

If the younger child is unable to explain or express verbally or is not willing, then that's absolutely acceptable and you must give the child the space to learn to trust the process and open up to you only when they are ready. Of course the other reason why they may not be able to explain or express the art verbally is because the piece simply isn't finished yet!

If you find the Theraplay times almost up and the child hasn't finished or you still need to continue working with the art, then you will need to store the work safely so the younger child can see and trust they can 'let go of it' and that you as the adult can be trusted to keep their art safe, which for the child means they may be testing you to see if you 'can be trusted with their sad and worrying memories.

It's therefore important to place or store the 'object' in a safe 'container'. For flat artwork, drawings, paintings etc. you can use a large A3 TRANSPARENT folder with a zip lock top.

It's important to allow the younger child the ability to place their art into the folder, and for you to then seal the folder, explaining that you will 'keep it safe' for them until they want to take it out, and to ask the child if they will 'allow or agree' to you doing this for them? If they say YES then store the folder somewhere safe, especially from other children, but in a place where the younger child knows where it is and can see it at home. They will then develop the trust in you not just as a person, an adult, but in your ability to keep their memories 'safe'. If they say NO then invite them to go and place it where they would like and explain they can look after it 'safely'. Be sure to explain at any point they can 'change their mind' and ask you to look after it safely when they feel ready to!

If the younger child has created a model or sculpture you should build an appropriate 'container' instead. Take a suitable sized box and cut out one side and the top. After the object has been placed into the 'container' use Clingfilm to seal the open sides, which still allows the child the ability to see inside the box, to ensure their work hasn't been tampered with, establishing that vital trust.

If the child wants to inspect or see their work at any time then you should allow them to do so by looking through the folder or box, which is why it must be transparent. Only take the art out when they are ready and willing and when there is time to add to it.

When the next play/art session is about to begin, collect the folder together and open it in front of the younger child, ask if 'you can take it out' again building on developing that trust. If not, then allow the child to do so, it's their work after all so why not!

Then begin the TheraPlay process again inviting the child to add to the art work, as they do ask the open questions as needed, gently guiding the Theraplay. This process may take just one session, or a few hours, days, weeks or even months, perseverance is absolutely essential. Take your time.

Remember as soon as the younger child can explain or express the art they have created you will be able to transition the OBJECT into the next step – 'FEEL'.

In order to do test this simply ask the younger child when they think about what they've created "WHERE CAN THEY FEEL THAT IN THEIR BODY"?

It may seem like a bizarre question for a young child but even at a young age they may know how to identify feelings in their bodies. FEEL is the very next step in the process for younger children, and adults and older children and we're going to look at that later on!

For younger children remember the first phase FIND while it might take longer to arrive at the memory, it is often much simpler than for adults and older children because we only find and work on just one memory at a time.

There is another much simpler technique that can help younger children 'FIND' instead of THERAPLAY, we can now use Animal Finger Puppets. You can buy these from local stores, online or have a go at making them yourselves from paper or even from just a sock if you are not in a position to buy any finger puppets or draw on you own finger.

Here is the selection I use in my clinics of around 4 puppets. It is helpful to give a young child a choice so they will always find one they would like to choose, but if you are only able to make a single sock puppet then play with this sock character often and build trust with the child and sock puppet and name it!

Your own ability to engage with the puppet is essential to make this real and engaging and fun for the child and for yourself!

I speak to the chosen finger puppet and start up a conversation with the child through the puppet having some fun engaging the child with the puppet. I can then ask the child to whisper what the memory is to the puppet, rather than tell me if they don't want to.

I then place the puppet to my ear as if the puppet speaks to me, but I pretend the puppet didn't hear what the child has just said, so I ask the child to whisper again to the puppet, and again I pretend the puppet cannot hear what the child is saying, so the next time I lean in and I listen to what the child says and ask them to speak up a bit or by this time they usually just shout it out!

When I hear the words I ensure I play out the 'puppet' has then told me and so we then have found the memory and we can move swiftly onto the next Step 2 - 'FEEL'.

Before we do move onto the next phase, here's quick simple re-cap of the Step ONE

Step 1 – Find

1. Identify traumatic memories by **MEMORY MAPPING or THERA PLAY** as above

2. For younger children use Finger Puppets or Theraplay

We usually at this stage detail a script for you to use, however the process can be as simple as asking one question, or if using Theraplay then it can take a number of days and there is no actual script necessary for this other than the guidelines above, which you can always refer to and read as you go along. I've still added a few scripted ideas to help you start this positively.

SCRIPT FOR YOUNGER CHILDREN – Step 1 FIND

As no detailed script is required for the phase one for young children you can simply ask this question...

"DO YOU REMEMBER WHEN ...."

(or)

"SHALL WE HAVE A LOOK AT YOUR LOVELY PICTURE" –

(Theraplay art work)

So let's move on to the 2nd phase for Adults, Older Children and Younger Children as we now look at 'FEEL'

Chapter 11

Step Two – 'FEEL'

Now we have identified the memory we are going to work on we are now going to allow the body to safely 'FEEL' the memory as if they were in that actual memory.

It's very important we do this, because for EMDR to work we need to ensure the mind is focused solely on that memory.

What happens when the mind focuses on that memory is that it will become fearful and the mind will put the body into the 'Fight or Flight' mode we've discussed and the brain will release the chemical CORTISOL, which induces ADRENALIN. Adrenalin is then pumped around the body by the heart at an increased rate, so the heart pumps or beats faster, and then the feeling of ANXIETY will kick in. We may feel anxiety in our Head, Chest or Stomach, sometimes in our arms, hands or legs. That's the FEELING we need to induce and isolate.

Why do we feel Anxiety?

When the body engages the 'Fight or Flight' response the purpose of the Adrenalin is to increase our ability to run away or fight that imaginary dinosaur we've talked about.

So the Adrenalin is pumped into areas of the body; the head so we can see and think better to evaluate our escape route (i.e through the trees) or attack strategy; or our arms and legs so we can run faster away, or to use the strength to fight the dinosaur with our spears - back in the days when we were cavemen, cavewomen and children. Anxiety goes all the way back to being a developed defence mechanism when we evolved from being Neanderthals into Homo sapiens.

So when the adrenalin pumps into these areas of the body above, it leaves the core of our body void or empty! This is why we often feel the anxiety in our gut or chest and why if we find we are continually in a state of 'Fight or Flight', because we are always so on edge or anxious (because we think there are dinosaurs everywhere coming to eat us) and if that feeling NEVER leaves us – we permanently suffer from being in a heightened state of alert, which is anxiety and panic.

In these cases we begin to develop disorders of the gut, IBS or eating disorders. It can make living with Autism, ADD, ADHD, Asperger, even harder when they experience sensory overload. Sometimes the Adrenalin is so overwhelming we cannot sit still, the increased levels in our legs or arms makes us fidget uncontrollably – our legs shake up and down, and our hands and fingers shake, perhaps so much we bite our finger nails or even the skin on our fingers. It's this feeling of sensory overload that can be most overwhelming, which is why it can cause the behaviour changes we've discussed, and it's why this 'feeling' is therefore very easy for the subject to 'find', even for a young child, as it's a pre-programmed automatic human response to what is ultimately being 'afraid' or fear!

Once we have isolated this feeling we know that the memory identified and recorded in the circle or the artwork is indeed causing the anxiety and we can then move onto the next step, which is the actual EASY EMDR treatment.

So let's begin.

This phase is almost exactly the same for each group of person - it doesn't matter if they are an Adult, Older or Younger Child when they think about what they've written in the circle (or for younger children told you directly or through a finger puppet or created with art therapy) the feeling is the same.

For Adults and Older Children

There's a little more to do as we are often working on multiple memories and we need to isolate each memory, whereas with younger children we only work on one memory at a time.

So you now have the Memory Map completed, make sure this is placed off to one side, but visible, we don't want any barriers in the way of the subject.

Pick up the Memory Map and show it to the subject and ask them to choose one of the circles to work on first.

TOP TIP - It's always best to work on one of the lower graded memories first to 'prove' to the subject EASY EMDR works!

Once they KNOW it works for themselves they will be far more inclined to proceed with the treatment of a more severe traumatic memory or the circles with the higher numbers.

The subject in a moment will use the same 4 TO 8 breath technique as we used to calm them, it is in fact the exact same technique we have already used to unblock the mind in the FIND stage.

In order to help isolate this feeling which is very simple ask the adult or older child (not younger child) to 'Close their Eyes' and then read the word or words written in the circle exactly as it is written.

You can say to them:

"Ok we're now going to work on the first memory so just close your eyes".

Then use the breathing technique 4 in 8 out, to relax the subject.

Ensure the subject has closed their eyes, then ask the subject to:

1. TAKE A DEEP BREATHE IN FILLING THE LUNGS AND SHOULDERS
2. When they are at the top of the breath say HOLD IT....HOLD IT...
3. AND EXHALE....MOUTH OPEN... SLOWLY BLOW ALL THE AIR OUT... THAT'S RIGHT.
4. Repeat steps 1-3 three times.
5. On the final breath out say "Now with your eyes closed continue to breath normally".

IT IS VERY IMPORTANT YOU DO NOT FORGET TO REMIND THE SUBJECT TO BREATHE NORMALY AFTERWARDS!!

Then say the words "I'm now going to mention a word or words to you, and when I do just allow your mind to go back in time to an early memory connected with whatever the word .... means to you".

SAY THE WORD/S.

Repeat the WORD/S.

Repeat "Just allow your mind to go back in time to an early memory connected with whatever the word/s .... means to you".

Ask them "JUST TELL ME WHEN YOU'RE THERE, WHEN YOU'RE IN THAT MEMORY".

They will either say "I'm there" or nod their head.

By repeating the word THREE times such repetition helps focus the mind deeper and deeper onto the memory of the trauma. Remember it doesn't matter what the word means to you – but say the word in a DELIBERATE SLOW manner with emphasis and a slight pause.

You can go to www.EASYEMDR.org to hear examples of how to use the tone, the inflection of your voice to deepen the subjects thought process.

Don't forget all the wording to be used for each and every step is included in the Step by Step guide found at the back of this book for easy quick reference.

Leave the subject to sit with their thoughts – say nothing more until they tell you "I'm there" or words to that effect".

As soon as they do ask them "WHERE CAN YOU FEEL THAT IN YOUR BODY"?

They will be able to answer out loud or sometimes they will just point or indicate with their hands in silence, either way they will tell you or point to an area in their body, the head, chest, stomach – all the places where we usually feel anxiety, or in uncommon cases the legs, arms, back, waist, hands or feet.

If they do speak they might say something like: "in my.....":

- Tummy
- Chest
- Head
- Neck
- Everywhere

YES they may even say EVERYWHERE.... or NOT at all!

Be prepared for whatever may be said, it doesn't really matter as long as the memory causes a physical reaction in the body.

If they can feel it GREAT - JOB DONE! Now it's onto the actual EMDR itself, but if the response is "Not At All" or "I can't Feel It" don't worry there's a very simple technique you can use called Image Projection and Enhancing a Memory to help the subject go into the memory, which we will look at later in this chapter on page 159.

Let's assume for now the subject CAN feel the anxiety, you must immediately ask them once again to grade the feeling on a scale of 0-10.

If it's a zero then the memory is NOT causing any anxiety. Similarly if the memory isn't causing any feeling in the body then that memory isn't the cause of the anxiety! This is one of the cross checks we carry out throughout to make sure the correct triggers of anxiety have been identified in the MEMORY MAPPING process.

If it's a zero or there's no feeling of anxiety present then simply move onto the next circle or group of circles.

If the subject can feel the anxiety, and can grade this on the scale of 0-10 as before for MEMORY MAPPING, zero being the lowest and 10 being the highest, then you are ready to move straight away to the next step and next chapter which is the EMDR treatment itself.

You will be able to see when you compare the RED number written in the MEMORY MAP to the actual number that the subject is 'feeling'. They should be the same or close to it, confirming the MEMORY MAP is accurate.

If they are very different, which can happen, for example the RED number on the MEMORY MAP is 10, but the feeling is 4, this is an indicator that the subjects mind is NOT fully engaged in the memory.

If this is the case there is a simple therapy you can use to deepen the engagement of the subject into the memory which will bring the numbers more into alignment - 'Image Projection and Enhancing a Memory'. It's important to ensure you do this to trigger the correct level of anxiety.

It's important to do so is because the mind has to be able to find ALL the memory not just the tip of the memory, or only that part will be treated and the remaining part of the unexposed memory will still be active and will still contribute to behaviour change.

It's like only finding the tip of an iceberg, we need to see the whole iceberg most of which is hidden under water to melt the whole iceberg!

Image Projection and Enhancing a Memory

The therapy you can use to deepen the engagement in the memory is very simple. Ensure your subject's eyes are still closed. Ask the subject to imagine a screen just in front of their mind, and invite them to project an image of the memory onto the screen. It can be a still image or a moving image. Then ask them to "reach out with their mind and find the dial marked COLOUR" and ask the subject to "turn the COLOUR of the image up, make the image brighter and clearer as if you are really there". The image will become clearer in the subjects mind. Then ask the subject to "reach out with their mind and find the dial marked VOLUME" and ask the subject to "turn the SOUND of the image up, make the sounds in the image LOUDER and CLEARER as if you are really there". The whole memory may then become clearer in the subjects mind.

Now ask the subject to check in again with the feeling, where is it now? Sometimes it moves into the gut or chest, and ask them "How bad is that feeling NOW on a scale of 0-10? Emphasise the word NOW. The memory should now be more in line with the original MEMORY MAP.

Be aware that by using this Projection Therapy you can often trigger a tearful emotional response. This is NOT something to be worried or afraid of, it just means so far you have completed the steps correctly, and this reaction is a positive one as all the memory has been 'exposed' or recalled, This is exactly where you want your subject to be. We have found the entire iceberg!

Move onto the next Step immediately without delay. The 'firework' has gone off with a BANG, now you need to FIZZLE it out fast!

If for any reason, which is highly unlikely and very uncommon the subject is becoming very distressed then use the SAFE PLACE process as before.

When working with Younger Children, this now becomes much easier from here on. As we discussed before you won't need to carry out the projection therapy with the child, we don't want to upset them, we just need to find the place where they can feel the anxiety and then start the EMDR.

It doesn't matter what the number is, as you never graded it before, we just accept that if a young child can actually feel anxiety then it doesn't matter how bad this is, we just need to DESENSITISE the child to that memory so they can effectively REPROCESS it, or remove it from their mind.

Here is the process for Adults or Older Children:

Visualisation Technique to Increase the 'FEELING'

1. Ask the subject to "IMAGINE THERE IS A SCREEN IN FRONT OF YOUR MIND, LIKE A TV OR CINEMA SCREEN".

2. Then after a few seconds ask them to "NOW PROJECT AN IMAGE OF THE MEMORY ONTO THE SCREEN, IT MIGHT BE A STILL OR A MOVING IMAGE", they should be able to do this – it's just visualisation and very simple.

3. Now again after a few seconds ask them to "NOW REACH OUT WITH YOUR MIND AND FIND THE DIAL MARKED VOLUME AND TURN THE SOUND UP – MAKE ALL THE SOUNDS IN THAT IMAGE LOUDER SO YOU CAN HEAR ABSOLUTELY EVERYTHING AS IF YOU WERE ACTUALLY THERE".

4. Now ask them to "NOW REACH OUT WITH YOUR MIND AND FIND THE DIAL MARKED COLOUR AND TURN THE COLOUR UP – MAKE ALL THE IMAGES BRIGHTER AND EVEN MORE COLOURFUL SO YOU CAN SEE ABSOLUTELY EVERYTHING AS IF YOU WERE ACTUALLY THERE".

5. Now ask the subject to "SLOWLY MOVE THE SCREEN TOWARD YOU, ALLOW THE IMAGE TO GET BIGGER AND BIGGER...".

6. Now ask the subject to "NOW STEP INTO THE IMAGE, AND SEE YOURSELF IN THAT IMAGE AS IF YOU WERE ACTUALLY THERE...".

7. Now ask them immediately: "WHERE CAN YOU FEEL THAT IN YOUR BODY NOW?".

As before they will be able to answer out loud or sometimes they will just point or indicate with their hands in silence, but if they do speak they might say something like: "in my...":

- Tummy
- Chest
- Head
- Neck

Or Everywhere.... or NOT at all again!

If it's NOT AT ALL again then there simply is NO FEAR or ANXIETY being triggered by this memory and you do not need to work on it with EMDR.

You can cross that one off the Memory Map and go onto choosing the next one together. You could ask them to cross it off to reinforce the result.

As soon as they **DO FEEL** the memory this is the Anxiety kicking in and this is exactly what we want to happen as we can now go onto the important **DESENSITISING** (the **D** in EMDR) of the subject to the memory which will allow them to effectively **'FORGET'**.

So you can now move onto the actual EMDR Treatment phase Step 3 - 'FOLLOW', which will REDUCE this feeling and thus TURN DOWN or DESENSITISE the subject to the memory.

SCRIPT FOR ADULTS AND OLDER CHILDREN - FEEL

OK WE ARE NOW GOING TO WORK ON THE FIRST MEMORY SO JUST CLOSE YOUR EYES.

BREATHE IN FILLING YOUR LUNGS AND SHOULDERS.

HOLD IT... HOLD IT...

BREATHE OUT SLOWLY EXHALE ALL THE AIR.

BREATHE IN FILLING YOUR LUNGS AND SHOULDERS.

HOLD IT... HOLD IT...

BREATHE OUT SLOWLY EXHALE ALL THE AIR.

BREATHE IN FILLING YOUR LUNGS AND SHOULDERS.

HOLD IT... HOLD IT... HOLD IT...

BREATHE OUT SLOWLY EXHALE ALL THE AIR.

I'M NOW GOING TO SAY A WORD TO YOU, AND WHEN I DO JUST ALLOW YOUR MIND TO GO ALL THE WAY BACK IN TIME TO AN EARLIER MEMORY CONNECTED WITH WHATEVER THE WORD ....(insert word from circle)........ MEANS TO YOU (say the words exactly as written in the circle).

(repeat the phrase again below)

JUST ALLOW YOUR MIND TO GO ALL THE WAY BACK IN TIME TO AN EARLIER MEMORY CONNECTED WITH WHATEVER THE WORD/S .... MEANS TO YOU.

(repeat again the words)

JUST TELL ME WHEN YOU'RE THERE, WHEN YOU'RE IN THAT MEMORY?

(they will either say "I'm there" or nod their head)

WHERE CAN YOU (emphasise 'feel') *FEEL* THAT IN YOUR BODY?

(they will either tell you or point to an area in their body)

HOW BAD IS THAT FEELING ON A SCALE OF 0-10.

(as soon as the subject grades the feeling, immediately compare the RED number written in the MEMORY MAP to the actual number that the subject is 'feeling'. They should be the same or within 3 points higher or lower – if so move onto the next Step 3 – 'FOLLOW' which is the EMDR treatment)

"KEEP YOUR EYES CLOSED".

(or)

(if the memory isn't causing any feeling in the body then that memory isn't the cause of the anxiety - move onto the VISUALISATION TECHNIQUE below which starts IMAGINE A SCREEN....)

(if they are very different this is an indicator that the subjects mind is not fully engaged – use the script below to deepen the engagement in the memory)

(ensure your subject's eyes are still closed)

IMAGINE A SCREEN JUST IN FRONT OF YOUR MIND.

NOW PROJECT AN IMAGE OF THE MEMORY ONTO THE SCREEN IT CAN BE A STILL IMAGE OR A MOVING IMAGE.

NOW REACH OUT WITH YOUR MIND AND FIND THE DIAL MARKED COLOUR AND TURN THE COLOUR OF THE IMAGE UP.

MAKE THE IMAGE BRIGHTER AND CLEARER AS IF YOU ARE ACTUALLY THERE.

(wait 10 seconds)

NOW REACH OUT WITH YOUR MIND AND FIND THE DIAL MARKED VOLUME AND TURN THE SOUND OF THE IMAGE UP.

MAKE THE IMAGE LOUDER AND CLEARER AS IF YOU ARE REALLY THERE SO YOU CAN HEAR ABSOLUTELY EVERYTHING.

WHERE CAN YOU FEEL THAT IN YOUR BODY *NOW*?

(emphasise the word NOW)

HOW BAD IS THAT FEELING ON A SCALE OF 0-10?

(the number should now be similar to the original MEMORY MAP)

(you can now move onto the EMDR Treatment phase Step 3 – 'FOLLOW', which will REDUCE this feeling and TURN DOWN or DESENSITISE the subject to the memory)

"KEEP YOUR EYES CLOSED".

For a younger child

Remember this phase is almost exactly the same for each group of person.

As soon as they tell you what the memory is just ask the child:

"WHERE CAN YOU FEEL THAT INSIDE YOUR BODY"?

This step is very quick and easy as younger children do not over think this.

SCRIPT FOR A YOUNGER CHILD

(as soon as they tell you what the memory is just ask the child...)

"WHERE CAN YOU FEEL THAT INSIDE YOUR BODY"?

"KEEP YOUR EYES CLOSED".

(you can now move onto the EMDR Treatment phase Step 3 – 'FOLLOW', which will REDUCE this feeling and TURN DOWN or DESENSITISE the subject to the memory)

Chapter 12

STEP THREE – 'FOLLOW'

EMDR Treatment Phase

So now we have arrived at the most important and exciting stage which is the actual EMDR treatment. Again I'm going to explain this process for Adults, then Older Children, then Younger Children as the process has variations for all based on the Adult process, so it's important you learn this first. Again there are FREE online tutorials at www.EASYEMDR.org.

Get ready now comes the MAGIC YOU'VE WAITED FOR!

Eye Movement Technique

You are now going to DESENSITISE your subject to the memory they are thinking about:

1. Make sure you're sat about 1.5 foot or 40 centimetres from the subjects' knees with you both sat on chairs facing each other at the same height. Make sure you set the chairs up before the subject even walks into the room. Your hands when raised must be the same height as the subject's eyes.

2. Whilst their eyes are CLOSED ready yourself quickly, and if needed you must be able to reach comfortably to tap their knees.

3. Hold your left hand up in the air palm turned up as if cradling their chin from a distance – it's a visual reminder for the subject to KEEP THEIR HEAD PERFECTLY STILL.

4. Now hold up your other hand with your first and second fingers pointing horizontally at the subjects eyes palm facing down, all other fingers tucked in. Take a close look at the image below to ensure you are holding your hands in the correct way.

Remember your subject will at this time be imagining a traumatic memory and we do not want nor need to prolong their emotions any more than is necessary so be ready to act IMMEDIATELY.

Please visit www.EASYMDR.org to see a demonstration if required.

5. Ask the subject to "OPEN YOUR EYES, KEEP YOUR HEAD STILL AND FOLLOW MY FINGERS LEFT AND RIGHT".

Now move your fingers slowly **LEFT** and **RIGHT** on an imaginary horizontal line, ensure the subject is FOLLOWING your fingers with their eyes, if not just say "FOLLOW MY FINGERS".

You may have to say this more than once as they may easily forget.

Concentrate on them following your fingers at an even speed not too slow or too fast, each full movement should only take about 1 second, count to yourself 1, 2, 1, 2, 1, 2 – move your fingers fully to the left of their vision and then fully to the right. Stay just inside their vision. Again take a look at the image above to ensure your hand movements are correct and they are moving their eyes, following your fingers all the way Left and Right.

6. Keep moving your fingers back and forth. As this happens the sensitivity or the feeling they had located relating to the memory they are still thinking of will start to reduce. It may take a few seconds or a few minutes or in rare cases 10 minutes. We are now going to help that memory reduce in sensitivity even faster!

7. Say to the subject whilst moving your fingers "KEEP FOCUSSING ON THAT OLD MEMORY AND THAT OLD FEELING AS IT STARTS TO COME ALL THE WAY DOWN". This is important to ensure they don't drift off into another memory, keep repeating this every few minutes as a reminder, there's no need to go over the top with repeating it. It's just a reminder.

8. You can help speed up the **DESENSITISATION** further by now saying "THE MORE IT REDUCES THE CALMER YOU FEEL, THE CALMER YOU FEEL THE MORE IT REDUCES AS YOUR MIND KNOWS EXACTLY WHERE IT NEEDS TO GO ON ITS OWN TO HEAL - DOESN'T IT?"

9. Now ask the subject "AS IT STARTS TO GO DOWN WHAT NUMBER WOULD YOU LIKE IT TO GO DOWN TO A... ZERO A ONE OR A TWO?" They will respond with a number, the method is to just keep going until that number is reached and then STOP.

10. How will you know when that magic number has been reached? Just ask! After about 10 hand movements ask the subject "FOCUS ON THAT OLD FEELING - WHAT HAS IT GONE DOWN TO NOW?" Prompt the subject to give you a number as before on the scale of 0-10 and you will BOTH see it has come down!

11. Keep moving your fingers from side to side and keep asking "WHAT HAS THE NUMBER GONE DOWN TO NOW?" It will decrease number by number or it may drop or decrease in 2's, 3's, 4's or drop even more rapidly. It really is THAT easy!

12. When you get to the desired number they have chosen just STOP and ask the subject to close their eyes.

Additional Sensory Techniques to Speed Up EMDR

So what if it doesn't come down? Keep Going! It Will!

Here are a few extra simple but incredibly effective techniques to speed up the EMDR or **FOLLOW** phase. They can also be used if a subject has a Visual Impairment, or struggles with focusing on following your fingers, this is especially helpful for people with ADD, ADHD, Asperger or Autism. EMDR has the exact same effect regardless if the subjects' eyes are **OPEN OR CLOSED** if you follow the additional techniques below:

If you find a subject is taking a little more time and the anxiety feeling is not reducing or is stuck, on any number then you can now increase the stimulation by adding **SOUND**! We know that **EM** is Eye Movement, this stimulates the left and right brain using the sense of sight, but you can also stimulate the left and right brain by just clicking your fingers as they move farthest right and farthest left as well, introducing **SOUND**.

As the subject follows your fingers which is **SIGHT** – now we have TWO senses being used; **CLICK LEFT... CICK RIGHT**.
You can also introduce a third sense **TOUCH** or if a subject has a Visual Impairment, or struggles with focusing on following your fingers. This is again especially helpful for people with ADD, ADHD, Asperger, Autism or even if undiagnosed anyone whose attention wanders. You can achieve this by **TAPPING** the subject's knees, ask them for their consent first of course!

Tap the LEFT and then RIGHT KNEE lightly with two fingers, but firm enough for the subject to feel the tap – you should be able to hear the tap slightly on the hollow knee. As the brain is effectively cross wired by tapping the left knee this will stimulate the right side of the brain, and vice versa for the right knee, it will stimulate the left side of the brain. TAP LEFT.... TAP RIGHT counting in your mind 1, 2, 1, 2, 1, 2 to establish the correct rhythm.

It is quite amazing to see the EMDR process have the exact same effect with the eyes closed – this really does feel like **MIND MAGIC!** Again the tapping rather than the eye movement will reduce the numbers, the feeling in the process is exactly the same and should be substituted as and when required. If the Eye Movement is taking too long then why not try using the **CLICKS** or **TAPPING** instead. Or just have fun and try it out any way!

You can use a combination of all three at any time in the same session – I do regularly – especially with children and we will come onto this in the sections that follow for Older and Younger Children. Invite the subject to FOLLOW YOUR FINGERS as you TAP so you TAP LEFT AND RIGHT as the subject also follows your fingers so their eyes also move LEFT and RIGHT using 2 senses at the same time, in fact as our knees are hollow when you tap they will also hear SOUND as if you were clicking so that's now 3 senses being used at the same time which speeds up the EMDR!

So if we can **TAP** with our eyes closed why is it called EMDR – which again is **EYE** Movement Desensitisation and Reprocessing?

The actual treatment relies on the bi-lateral stimulation of the brain and not just the eyes so any sense will work; SIGHT, SOUND, or TOUCH. Therefore it should and is in fact called:

BLS or BI-LATERAL STIMULATION DESENSITISATION & REPROCESSING but that longer acronym spells **BLSDR** a complex abbreviation and not ideally suitable for a medical treatment and so the single stimulation abbreviation EMDR was born as BLS was too long!

SCRIPT FOR ADULTS- FOLLOW

OPEN YOUR EYES, KEEP YOUR HEAD STILL – AND FOLLOW MY FINGERS LEFT AND RIGHT.

KEEP FOLLOWING MY FINGERS.

(you may have to say this more than once as they may easily forget).

KEEP FOCUSSING ON THAT OLD MEMORY AND THAT OLD FEELING AS IT STARTS TO COME ALL THE WAY DOWN.

WHAT NUMBER WOULD YOU LIKE IT TO GO DOWN TO A... ZERO, A ONE, OR A TWO?

KEEP FOCUSSING ON THAT OLD MEMORY AND THAT OLD FEELING AS IT STARTS TO COME ALL THE WAY DOWN.

THE MORE IT COMES DOWN THE CALMER YOU FEEL, THE CALMER YOU FEEL THE MORE IT COMES DOWN AS YOUR MIND KNOWS EXACTLY WHAT IT NEEDS TO FIND TO HEAL DOESN'T IT?

(keep moving fingers with eyes following for approx. 10 seconds or if the eyes blink this is a good indicator the number has gone down so ask again...)

KEEP FOCUSING ON THAT OLD MEMORY AND THAT OLD FEELING - WHAT NUMBER HAS IT COME DOWN TO NOW?

(they will respond with a number, the method is to just keep going moving your fingers with eyes following until that number comes all the way down to the required number)

KEEP FOCUSING ON THAT OLD MEMORY AND THAT OLD FEELING - WHAT NUMBER HAS IT COME DOWN TO NOW?

(it will decrease number by number or it may drop or decrease in 2's, 3's, 4's or drop even more rapidly)

HUM HUM… HUM HUM… HUM HUM.

(keep acknowledging without words you are still paying attention)

(when they get close to the desired number say…)

AND FINALLY……. LET GO! WHAT'S IT COME DOWN TO NOW?

(STOP when they say TWO, ONE or ZERO whatever number they choose)

CLOSE YOUR EYES.

Now you can move onto the fourth and final Step 4 – 'FORGET' for ADULTS.

Step 3 – FOLLOW for OLDER CHILDREN

The process is the exact same as for the adults but now we are going to use **MIND MAGIC** again – tell the child we are now going to help them FORGET this memory by using a MAGIC spell, and to do this we use a MAGIC Wand to almost RUB OUT the memory by going BACK & FORTH – LEFT to RIGHT with the wand. The more the wand moves the more the memory fades as it comes down until is gone! Just follow the exact same procedure for adults except you use a wand rather than your fingers! It couldn't be simpler, just remind them to keep following the wand!

Again if they do not respond well to the wand movements then you can switch to the other stimulus by taping their knees. I explain to children "I'm like a very powerful wizard and sometimes I don't need to use a wand – I can do magic with my HANDS just like many witches and wizards we see on TV and film, and if I use my hands to tap your knees it's the same spell as using a magic wand!".

CAUTION: REMEMBER if you are treating a child and you are not their legal guardian then you must ensure the child and your session is always supervised by a responsible adult.

You must ALWAYS obtain the consent of the adult and the child to touch them by tapping their knees. This is what we call consent to appropriate touching. Even if the responsible adult or guardian agrees, even if they are your own child or family member it is ALWAYS appropriate and necessary to ask the child, respect their wishes.

There may be very good reasons why they do not want to be touched and their wishes must always be respected. We NEVER force a child or even an adult for that matter it is their human right to say NO. If they do say NO you can explain by demonstrating on yourself how you will just ONLY tap their knees lightly. This may help the child to make an informed decision, you are not attempting to persuade them to agree to something they do not want.

Again if they say no then it's a NO and you will have to revert to eye movement with clicking where possible.

So the last thing we asked our subject to do was "KEEP YOUR EYES CLOSED", let's pick up from there on what we are now going to do next.

Remember where you are now already in the process; the child would have just closed their eyes and would have connected to the memory and graded the feeling.

1. Now ask the child to "OPEN YOUR EYES" and then use the wand to track the eyes left and right, say "FOLLOW THE WAND WITH YOUR EYES, KEEP YOUR HEAD STILL" as the memory sensitivity again reduces as per the adult version.

2. Keep moving the wand and keep checking in with where the feeling is until it has come down to zero or the number the child has chosen. Depending on age you can chose to not give the child the choice of number, usually older children will have more developed minds that can make this choice, for slightly younger minds it will acceptable to just keep reducing until **"it's gone!"**.

3. As soon as the memory has GONE tell the child to "CLOSE YOUR EYES" and move onto Step 4 – 'FORGET'.

SCRIPT FOR OLDER CHILDREN - FOLLOW

OPEN YOUR EYES, KEEP YOUR HEAD STILL – AND FOLLOW THE WAND LEFT AND RIGHT.

KEEP FOLLOWING THE WAND.

(you may have to say this more than once as they may easily forget)

KEEP FOCUSSING ON THAT OLD MEMORY AND THAT OLD FEELING AS IT STARTS TO COME ALL THE WAY DOWN.

WHAT NUMBER WOULD YOU LIKE IT TO GO DOWN TO A... ZERO, A ONE, OR A TWO?

KEEP FOCUSSING ON THAT OLD MEMORY AND THAT OLD FEELING AS IT STARTS TO COME ALL THE WAY DOWN.

THE MORE IT COMES DOWN THE CALMER YOU FEEL, THE CALMER YOU FEEL THE MORE IT COMES DOWN.

(keep moving wand with eyes following for approx. 10 seconds or if the eyes blink this is a good indicator the number has gone down so ask again...)

KEEP FOCUSING ON THAT OLD MEMORY AND THAT OLD FEELING - WHAT NUMBER HAS IT COME DOWN TO NOW?

(they will respond with a number, the method is to just keep going moving your wand with eyes following until that number comes all the way down to the required number)

KEEP FOCUSING ON THAT OLD MEMORY AND THAT OLD FEELING - WHAT NUMBER HAS IT COME DOWN TO NOW?

(it will decrease number by number or it may drop or decrease in 2's, 3's, 4's or drop even more rapidly)

HUM HUM... HUM HUM... HUM HUM.

(keep acknowledging without words you are still paying attention, when they get close to the desired number say...)

AND FINALLY....... LET GO! WHAT'S IT COME DOWN TO NOW?

(STOP when they say TWO, ONE or ZERO whatever number they choose)

CLOSE YOUR EYES.

Now you can move onto the fourth and final phase Step 4 – 'FORGET'.

Step 3 – Follow for Younger Children – Using Finger Puppets

1. The child has already chosen a Finger Puppet, so ask the child to follow with their eyes the DOG, MOUSE, CAT which ever they have chosen. It is always helpful to have another adult on standby as very often the child will move their head not their eyes.

   The other adult assisting can kneel behind the child and gently with the open palms of their hands on either side of the child's head behind the ears just hold the head very gently to stop movement. This ensures only the child's eyes move following the puppet creating the bi-lateral stimulation (BLS) needed.

2. As the child is reminded to keep focusing on the memory of the picture or object reflecting the trauma, just ask them if they can still 'feel it' don't worry about what number it is as it will come down very quickly.

3. Finally ask them to tell you when it's 'GONE'. They usually shout that out!

That's it! For younger children the EMDR is very easy and very quick to take effect, the challenge is finding the trauma. You can recheck the memory again the next time you chose to work together.

SCRIPT FOR YOUNGER CHILDREN – FOLLOW

OPEN YOUR EYES.

AND NOW FOLLOW THE .... (use the name of the finger puppet dog, cat, mouse etc).

KEEP THINKING OF THAT MEMORY OF .... (name the memory they used).

KEEP FOLLOWING THE .... (finger puppet name).

IF YOU CAN STILL 'FEEL IT' DON'T WORRY IT WILL START TO GO AWAY.

KEEP THINKING OF THAT MEMORY OF .... (name the memory they used).

KEEP FOLLOWING THE .... (finger puppet name).

IF YOU CAN STILL 'FEEL IT' DON'T WORRY IT WILL KEEP GOING AWAY UNTIL IT'S......GONE.

JUST TELL ME WHEN IT'S GONE?

Once the feeling has GONE at this stage the child may want to go off and play and that's more than ok, it's probably quiet new to them, but with continued use this can be built into the weekly family routine so it becomes normal and what a great way to teach and prepare your child for those troublesome teenage years ahead!

If they do want to jump up and go off happy do let them as there is no real need to check back in with the child if it has gone at this point, you can do this another day, and so they will have already completed the final and fourth Step – 'FORGET'!

We need not do any more just yet. You can revisit the subject the next time you work together INDIRECTLY or DIRECTLY with the THERAPLAY, perhaps in a few days (as remember we always leave it at least 48 hours).

Perhaps the next time you DIRECT them to think about how they now feel they might draw or create a picture that is different, perhaps drawing a more positive perspective from a child's point of view. But if the child is still sat down waiting patiently and happy to still engage or take part then you can indeed now go back and just check that it has gone – and you can do this by now moving onto the fourth and final Step for younger children – 'FORGET'.

If you are still experiencing difficulty after much time spent you can where available or affordable choose to seek a professional therapist's advice or help, but I don't want to instantly set you up for failure to say this WILL happen, it's more than likely you might not need to. If you do then remember that's what we as professional therapists are here for too.

If you do not have access to professional therapy then there is no harm in just revisiting the protocols above again and again even if it means leaving therapy until their minds have developed a little further.

If professional help is not available then do not give up, you have nothing to lose but everything to gain from this EASY EMDR system no matter how long it may take.

Chapter 13

Step 4 – 'FORGET'

'Forget' for Adults

Remember we have left the subject with their eyes closed and they have just followed your fingers, or your hands tapping on their knees to desensitise or reduce the level of anxiety connected to the memory they were thinking about to a two, one or zero. Now we are going to move onto the last and final step.

1. Ask the subject to immediately OPEN THEIR EYES and now start asking them questions designed to CONFUSE them. You can use the ones from the list below or make up your own as you go along as I often do! It doesn't matter what you ask them as long as it is NOT related to the memory or subject or trauma, keep it light and fun but design the questions to confuse. As soon as they are confused and you will see this then TELL them to CLOSE THEIR EYES – don't necessarily wait for any answer!

Why do we do this? In order to make sure the treatment works we need to ensure the subject stops thinking about the memory entirely (before we go back to memory after to test it has worked) and we do this by what is referred to as 'BREAKING STATE'.

Suggested ideas for breaking state questions:

1. List the colours of the rainbow in alphabetical order GO!
2. What's the opposite of Purple?
3. What is paper made from?
4. What's the fourth planet from the moon?
5. Spell Ballerina with no vowels?
6. What's the heaviest animal in the world?
7. What's the highest mountain in the world?
8. What's the smallest mountain in the world?
9. What was your budgies name again?
10. What's the fastest train in the world?
11. What's the slowest train in the world?
12. Give me your mobile telephone number backwards?
13. Give me your car registration backwards?
14. What is the chemical symbol for Gold?
15. What is water made up of?
16. How many fathoms in a mile?
17. What's the largest animal in the world?
18. Spell Pseudonym?
19. What is glass made from?
20. Name three flowers that are Yellow?
21. Name a flower that's Green?

The list can go on and on, just ask anything that's a bit hard to answer no matter the intellect of the person, remember it's not designed to test IQ it's designed to confuse so the memory is disregarded.

2. So you've seen the subject is confused and you've TOLD them to "CLOSE YOUR EYES", now immediately ask them to go back to the OLD MEMORY and the OLD FEELING – it's very important to add the word OLD here so its recognised as past tense.

3. You can use these words "NOW GO BACK TO THE **OLD** MEMORY AND FOCUS ON THAT **OLD** FEELING AND TELL ME IF THE **OLD** FEELING IT STILL THERE, HAS IT GONE, OR IS IT THERE JUST A LITTLE BIT?"

4. If it's gone they will appear very happy and probably somewhat shocked and pleased. The first time the realisation that this terrible trauma has finally gone can be liberating yet sometimes confusing. Smile and make them feel proud of what they have just achieved, give them praise, a sincere "well done" goes a long way here or say "Welcome to the EMDR CLUB"!

5. Once this memory has been resolved then just go back to the Memory Map and start the whole process again.

6. If the feeling is still there JUST A LITTLE BIT then ask them "WHAT IS JUST A LITTLE BIT ON THE SCALE OF 0-10?" If it is a 1 or a 2 Ask them "ARE YOU ARE OK WITH THAT" – if YES stop, if NOT follow the steps below:

7. If it is a 3 or higher the EMDR protocol requires this to be resolved a little more so just follow the steps below:

8. If the FEELING is still there, ask the subject again "WHERE CAN YOU FEEL IT IN YOUR BODY?". You see we are just repeating the process exactly as we have done before, as it is quite common for a feeling to still be there, but this time it will probably be lower. Start the process again as before, ask them to GRADE THE FEELING ON A SCALE OF 0-10, and then hold up your hands, get ready and ask them to open their eyes and begin the EMDR again, it will go down again and then:

9. Break State using the same process as above, ask them to refocus on the old memory and the old feeling and the feeling this time may have finally gone! Or if it's there just a bit again then start the process again.

10. Keep going chipping away at the feeling, bringing the sensitivity down and rechecking and chip away a bit more etc. until its finally gone.

11. Different people respond differently to EMDR so be prepared for it to drop and go away in one go, and equally be prepared for it to take a few go's, both are very common. But what is always common is that it WILL... no matter how long it takes to come down... **IT WILL COME DOWN!**

Evaluating the Success

So now finally the MIND MAGIC has worked is time to make sure! Here is a really simple question to ask. In order to do so ask the subject to again close their eyes.

Tell the subject "NOW THAT THE FEELING HAS GONE / OR HAS COME DOWN TO THE LOW NUMBER YOU CHOSE, HOW GOOD DOES THAT NOW FEEL ON A NEW SCALE? THE NEW SCALE IS NOW 1-7, 1 BEING OK, 7 BEING FANTASTIC?"

Wait for the answer, which to be deemed successful should be 5, 6 or 7. If it is 5 or higher congratulate them. Why not ask them how they now feel?

If it is a lower number this is an indication the trauma may not be resolved. If the subject has multiple trauma as seen by many circles on their memory map, then at first it may take a few memories to be resolved, so you can always go back and re check this later after you've had a few 5's, 6's 7's, which is common.

If the number is still low then ask the subject why they feel it hasn't been resolved or why it doesn't feel that good, ask them to write a word describing this in a new circle on their existing memory map and work on this with the EMDR 4 step process and repeat until it is resolved.

Remember there are Step by Step simple guides to use at the end of this book or downloadable from www.EASYEMDR.org.

SCRIPT FOR ADULTS – 'FORGET'

OPEN YOUR EYES.

(ask 2 or 3 questions to confuse from the list below or make up your own)

LIST THE COLOURS OF THE RAINBOW IN ALPHABETICAL ORDER – GO!
WHAT'S THE OPPOSITE OF PURPLE?
WHAT IS PAPER MADE FROM?
WHAT'S THE FOURTH PLANET FROM THE MOON?
SPELL BALLERINA WITH NO VOWELS?
WHAT'S THE HEAVIEST ANIMAL IN THE WORLD?
WHAT'S THE HIGHEST MOUNTAIN IN THE WORLD?
WHAT'S THE SMALLEST MOUNTAIN IN THE WORLD?
WHAT'S THE FASTEST TRAIN IN THE WORLD?
WHAT'S THE SLOWEST TRAIN IN THE WORLD?
GIVE ME YOUR MOBILE NUMBER BACKWARDS?
GIVE ME YOUR CAR REGISTRATION BACKWARDS?
WHAT IS THE CHEMICAL SYMBOL FOR GOLD?
WHAT IS WATER MADE UP OF?
HOW MANY FATHOMS IN A MILE?
WHAT'S THE LARGEST ANIMAL IN THE WORLD?
WHAT IS GLASS MADE FROM?
NAME THREE FLOWERS THAT ARE YELLOW?
NAME A FLOWER THAT'S GREEN?

(as soon as they are confused or you've asked 3 questions...)

CLOSE YOUR EYES.

GO BACK TO THE **OLD** MEMORY AND FOCUS ON THAT **OLD** FEELING AND TELL ME IF THE OLD **FEELING** IS STILL THERE, HAS IT GONE, OR IS IT THERE JUST A LITTLE BIT?

(if the feeling is still there *JUST A LITTLE BIT* then ask them...)

WHAT IS JUST A LITTLE BIT ON THE SCALE OF 0-10?".

(if it's a 1 or a 2 ask them....)

ARE YOU ARE OK WITH THAT?

(if YES stop and jump ahead to Evaluating Success at the bottom of the next page, if NOT follow the steps below)

(or)

(if it's a ZERO jump ahead to Evaluating Success at the bottom of the next page)

(or)

(if it's a 3 or higher follow the steps below and ask the subject...)

WHERE CAN YOU FEEL IT IN YOUR BODY?

(wait for the reply)

HOW MUCH ON A SCALE OF 0-10?

(wait for the reply and hold up your fingers ready to restart again)

OPEN YOUR EYES.

(begin the phase three FOLLOW EMDR process again, it will go down again)
(Break State using different questions as above, ask them to refocus on the old memory and the old feeling, which this time may have finally gone! Or if it's there just a bit again then start the process again)

Keep going chipping away at the feeling, bringing the sensitivity down and rechecking and chip away a bit more etc. until its finally gone.

Evaluating the success

NOW THAT THE FEELING HAS GONE / OR HAS COME DOWN TO THE LOW NUMBER YOU CHOSE, HOW GOOD DOES THAT NOW FEEL ON A NEW SCALE OF ONE TO SEVEN, ONE BEING OK, SEVEN BEING FANTASTIC?

(wait for the answer successful should be 5, 6 or 7 - if it's 5 or higher congratulate them - why not ask them...)

HOW DO YOU NOW FEEL?

(if it's a number 4 or lower this indicates trauma may not be resolved)

(ask the subject)

WHY DO YOU FEEL IT HASN'T BEEN RESOLVED, WHY DOESN'T IT FEEL THAT GOOD?

(wait for the reply)

OK SO NOW WRITE ONE WORD DESCRIBING THIS IN A NEW CIRCLE ON YOUR EXISTING MEMORY MAP.

(work on this now and jump back to phase 2 FEEL and repeat until it is resolved)

Once this has been resolved then just go back to the Memory Map and start the whole process again)

Step 4 – FORGET for Older Children – Using Magic

Remember we have left the child with their eyes closed and they have just followed the wand or your fingers or your hands tapping on their knees to desensitise or reduce the level of anxiety connected to the memory they were thinking about to a two, one or zero. Now we are going to move onto the last and final step.

1. Ask the child to immediately open their eyes and now start asking them questions designed to CONFUSE them. You can use the ones from the list below or make up your own as you go along as I often do, depending on what the child is likely to be aware, which as a parent or guardian or friend you should have some idea of, if not then just ask a few questions before starting the treatment.

It doesn't matter what you ask them as long as it is NOT related to the memory or subject or trauma, keep it light and fun but design the questions to confuse. As soon as they are confused and you will see this then TELL them to close their eyes.

Why do we do this? In order to again make sure the treatment works we need to ensure the child stops thinking about the memory entirely (before we go back to the memory after to test it has worked) and we do this by what is termed as BREAKING STATE in the same way as for adults.

Example Breaking State Questions for Older Children:

1. What colour is Green & Blue mixed together?
2. What is an Apple crossed with an Orange?
3. What is a bridge over a railway called?
4. How many spots does a Lady Bird have?

Any questions are acceptable just keep them fun.

2. Once the child is confused – or sometimes even laughs! tell them to "CLOSE YOUR EYES" again!

3. Attempt to Re-trigger the memory as above using the adult step by step process. If it has not gone completely or is still there more than a 2 or higher then repeat the eye tracking with the wand.

4. When the feeling has finally 'gone' move onto the next memory and begin the entire process again.

Evaluating the Success

So now finally the MIND MAGIC has worked is time to make sure! Here is a really simple question to ask. In order to do so ask the child to again close their eyes.

Tell the child "NOW THAT THE FEELING HAS GONE / OR HAS COME DOWN TO THE LOW NUMBER YOU CHOSE, HOW GOOD DOES THAT NOW FEEL ON A NEW SCALE? THE NEW SCALE IS NOW 1-7, 1 BEING OK, 7 BEING FANTASTIC!?"

Wait for the answer which to be deemed successful should be 5, 6 or 7. If it is 5 or higher congratulate them. Why not ask them how they now feel?

If it is a lower number this is an indication the trauma may not be resolved.

If the child has multiple trauma as seen by many circles on their memory map, then at first it may take a few memories to be resolved. You can always go back and re check this later after you've had a few 5's, 6's or 7's, which is common.

If the number is still low then ask the subject why they feel it hasn't been resolved or why it doesn't feel that good?

Ask them to write a word describing this in a new circle on their existing memory map and work on this with the EMDR 4 step process and repeat until it is resolved.

SCRIPT FOR OLDER CHILDREN – 'FORGET'

OPEN YOUR EYES

(ask 2 or 3 questions to confuse from the list below or make up your own)

WHAT COLOUR IS GREEN & BLUE MIXED TOGETHER?
WHAT IS AN APPLE CROSSED WITH AN ORANGE?
WHAT IS A BRIDGE OVER A RAILWAY CALLED?
HOW MANY SPOTS DOES A LADY BIRD HAVE?

(as soon as they are confused or you've asked 3 questions...)

CLOSE YOUR EYES

GO BACK TO THE **OLD** MEMORY AND FOCUS ON THAT **OLD** FEELING AND TELL ME IF THE OLD **FEELING** IS STILL THERE, HAS IT GONE, OR IS IT THERE JUST A LITTLE BIT?

(if the feeling is still there *JUST A LITTLE BIT* then ask them...)

WHAT IS JUST A LITTLE BIT ON THE SCALE OF 0-10?"

(if it's a 1 or a 2 ask them....

ARE YOU ARE OK WITH THAT?

(if YES stop and jump ahead to Evaluating Success at the bottom of the page, if NOT follow the steps below)

(or)

(if it's a ZERO jump ahead to Evaluating Success at the bottom of the page)

(or)

(if it's a 3 or higher follow the steps below and ask the subject...)

WHERE CAN YOU FEEL IT IN YOUR BODY?

(wait for the reply)

HOW MUCH ON A SCALE OF 0-10?

(wait for the reply and hold up the wand or fingers ready to restart again from the phase three 'FOLLOW' EMDR process)

OPEN YOUR EYES.

(begin again, it will go down again, ask Break State questions using different questions as above, ask them to refocus on the old memory and the old feeling and the feeling this time may have finally gone - or if it's there just a bit again then start the process again)

Keep going chipping away at the feeling, bringing the sensitivity down and rechecking and chip away a bit more etc. until its finally gone.

(evaluating the success)

NOW THAT THE FEELING HAS GONE / OR HAS COME DOWN TO THE LOW NUMBER YOU CHOSE, HOW GOOD DOES THAT NOW FEEL ON A NEW SCALE OF ONE TO SEVEN, ONE BEING OK, SEVEN BEING FANTASTIC!?

(wait for the answer - success should be 5, 6 or 7 - if it's 5 or higher congratulate them – and why not now ask them...)

HOW DO YOU NOW FEEL?

(if it's a number 4 or lower this indicates trauma may not be resolved)

(ask the subject)

WHY DO YOU FEEL IT HASN'T BEEN RESOLVED, WHY DOESN'T IT FEEL THAT GOOD?

(wait for the reply)

OK SO NOW WRITE ONE WORD DESCRIBING THIS IN A NEW CIRCLE ON YOUR EXISTING MEMORY MAP

(work on this now and jump back to phase 2 FEEL and repeat until it is resolved)

(once this has been resolved then just go back to the Memory Map and start the whole process again)

Step 4 – FORGET For Younger Children

Remember the younger child may not need this phase as they may have already vanished excited to go and play! But if they are still engaged they will be sat in front of you with their EYES CLOSED, which is where we will pick up from.

Ask the child to open their eyes and follow the simple steps below:

1. Break State by asking very simple questions such as:

    Where do Fish live?
    What noise does a fire engine make?
    What's your favourite sweet?

2. Once they have answered you can ask them to "NOW TRY AND GO BACK TO THE OLD FEELING AND SEE IF IT'S THERE OR HAS IT GONE!" You are attempting to re trigger the memory again in the same way as for Older Children and Adults.

3. When the feeling has finally 'GONE' remove the finger puppet quickly and say YES LOOK ITS GONE! Removing the puppet reinforces the END, this is very important for a child to know. Praise the child and say WELL DONE! Tell them how good they have been.

4. If it's not gone completely or if it's more than a 2 or higher then go back to the memory and repeat the eye tracking with the finger puppet.

5. Once it has finally gone allow the child to move onto something completely different – "SHALL WE GO AND PLAY NOW?"

6. After a few days - move onto the next memory and begin the entire process again allowing at least 2 days to pass.

SCRIPT FOR YOUNGER CHILDREN – 'FORGET'

OPEN YOUR EYES.

(break state by asking very simple questions such as:)

WHERE DO FISH LIVE?
WHAT NOISE DOES A FIRE ENGINE MAKE?
WHAT'S YOUR FAVOURITE SWEET?

(wait for the reply)

NOW TRY AND GO BACK TO THE OLD FEELING AND SEE IF IT'S THERE OR HAS IT GONE?

(wait for the reply - when feeling has finally 'GONE' remove finger puppet quickly and say...)

YES LOOK IT'S GONE!

WELL DONE! YOU'VE BEEN REALLY GOOD - SHALL WE GO AND PLAY NOW?

(if not gone completely or a 2 or higher then go back to memory and repeat eye tracking with finger puppet)

After a few days you can move onto the next memory and begin the entire process again allowing at least 2 days to pass.

Chapter 14

After EMDR – What Next?

So now finally the MIND MAGIC has worked it is time to make sure! Here is a really simple question to ask. In order to do so ask the subject to again close their eyes.

Ask the subject:

"NOW THAT THE ALL THOSE FEELINGS HAVE GONE HOW GOOD DO YOU NOW FEEL?"

"DO YOU FEEL JUST OK, REALLY GOOD OR FANTASTIC!?"

If it's just OK then this is an indication the trauma may not be fully resolved, so always go back and re check this later after a few days – it's what we call a REVIEW and if the feeling or memory is still there you can work on this with the EASY EMDR 4 step process again and repeat until it is resolved.

To help us with this we are now going to look at what we call the 'Expected Outcomes'.

EMDR continues to still work for a further one to two days after treatment so expect the feelings to improve even more.

- Sleep should start to restore
- Anxiety should start to reduce or even resolve completely
- Levels of Stress should reduce
- Subjects should start to feel much happier, calmer, more at peace
- Stronger and more able to deal with day to day life
- Certain fears if worked on may have resolved fully
- Reports of feeling 'lighter' are extremely common

Why? Because after EMDR resolves the locked in traumas the subject goes from having Post Traumatic Stress to experiencing the elation of the direct opposite which is called **Post Traumatic GROWTH!**

This is an incredibly powerful state of mind to be in and one that can be capitalised upon by finally doing the things and taking on the challenges that were prevented by the weight of stress and anxiety and trauma bearing down on the subject's will power and energy and interest levels.

It may be that after a few days some residual memories come back, tis is very common, and so you just revisit the EMDR process again. You just keep going again and again until full resolution is finally achieved. But if in a few days NO memories come back then this is Full Resolution, and can be just as common.

Do not give up hope it will happen even if it does take up to the six minimum or recommended full session lengths of 12 (according to the W.H.O.), however in my extensive experience I see this change in just 2 to 4 sessions although yes for some people with very complex trauma with deep rooted physical manifestations or actual symptoms like pain from anxiety or IBS, it may indeed take up to the 12 sessions. The most I've ever used though is 11.

It is important to understand that for very complex cases where a full resolution cannot be achieved by using EASY EMDR at home, it is advisable to seek the further help from a clinical practitioner who specialises in EMDR.

However if you cannot afford the costs of ongoing treatment then having some resolution with using this book will be far better than having none what so ever. We recognise in some areas further help may not even exist.

What if it doesn't work completely? Could you imagine what it would feel like if you just had 50% more mental capacity to deal with the everyday stress of life, or higher? That might be better than again nothing! This is why EASY EMDR is such an essential front line tool in the treatment of the mental health issues and disorders at home or in the community. In my experience I am yet to come across a single person EMDR does not work for fully, unless they are not engaged in the process. This can be due to simple lack of will or because of diseases like Alzheimer's where the subject cannot 'find' memories.

So are there any side effects to be concerned about? The answer is NO! There are no known reported side effects of EMDR.

However sometimes subjects report feeling tired afterwards, this is not a side effect of EMDR this is a perfectly reasonable experience to have after moving your eyes left to right for an hour or two and concentrating hard!

In rare cases subjects can wake the next day feeling somewhat hazy or blank, or feeling like they do not know what to do with their life.

This again is not a side effect of EMDR, it is again a perfectly reasonable feeling after having so much trauma and bad memories stored in the mind that when it's suddenly all gone, if it's been there for as long as the subject can remember, then this feeling of emptiness can actually be quite daunting.

But it is in relative terms a much safer and better space to be in, perhaps a nice challenge to have, although to the subject it may not feel like this at all.

So this is where ongoing therapy such as CBT or Counselling or even better MINDFULNESS CAN help to build on the success of the EASY EMDR treatment and we can look at what is best suited to follow EMDR later on.

So now you are ready to begin treating adults and children if you've read this through and had some practice along the way.

If you have a small group of friends or parents, perhaps you could all help treat each other in a mini community home clinic held over coffee mornings? The possibilities now you are ready to go are endless.

I've broken down and grouped the different phase's step by step and by subject group of adult, older and younger children to help you learn and practice the techniques and reinforce how EASY EMDR actually is.

In the chapters that follow I've grouped all the scripts to help you run through a whole session from start to finish, for an adult, older or younger child, so you don't have to flick through the book for ease or reference.

I've also added some simple illustrations to help explain the process to your subjects in an easy to explain format, no matter what language they speak they should help to bridge a language barrier.

We've also added some tips on how to actually best perform a session. The main thing to remember is EMDR IS EASY so just get stuck in and if you get it a bit wrong just go back and correct yourself you cannot do any harm!

Chapter 15

Conduct a Session for Adults

(with full scripts & illustrations)

The more you practice with EMDR the easier you will be able to recall and deliver the treatment, perhaps it will become such second nature that in time you won't even need to refer to the scripts below, which is often the case, after just a few weeks I found I didn't.

Please don't worry if you don't get the words exactly correct, you can just go back over them and correct yourself, it will not affect the treatment at home at all. Remember you are doing this for FREE so no one's paying you, and you can't do any harm.

Whatever you do as long as you turn down or desensitise the feelings of anxiety it's going to work! Don't be afraid just GO FOR IT – the Mind Magic awaits!

Before starting the 4 step EASY EMDR process it may be helpful, if this is the first time the subject is experiencing EMDR, that you go back to the Anxiety Graph and use the images and explanations there to talk about how anxiety develops explaining it is the triggers, the memories of what is upsetting the subject or the traumas, that have accumulated to build the feeling and symptoms of anxiety and the associated disorders.

You can then explain why it's important to then work out what the triggers actually are, the memories or the traumas of what is upsetting for the subject, and how this can now be done quickly and easily with talking about them – or verbalising them.

Once they understand the reason why they are about to work out or 'FIND' the building blocks of their anxiety, you can then move onto the MEMORY MAPPING process and script below.

To use the scripts SAY everything in CAPITAL LETTERS, the lowercase words in brackets are reminders or simple instructions to keep you on track. Refer the subject to the simple illustrations provided over the page on each page for each step if helpful:

(space intentionally left blank)

SCRIPTS & ILLUSTRATIONS - FOR ADULTS

STEP 1 – FIND (ADULTS)

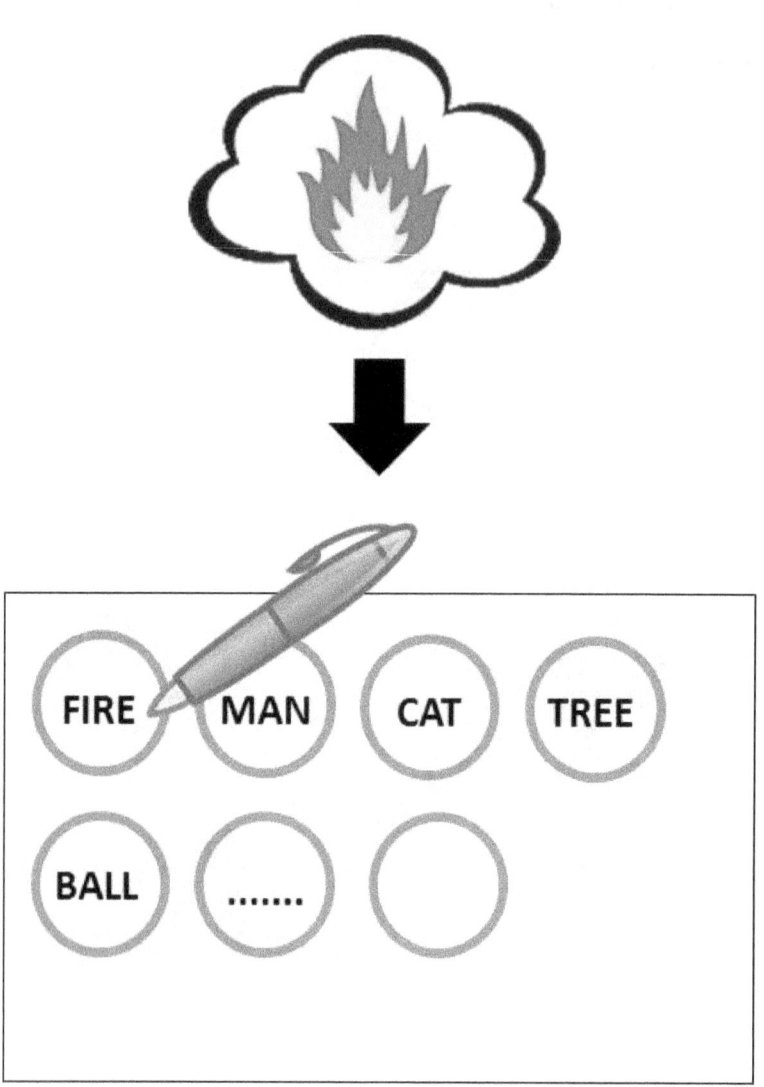

STEP 2 – FEEL (ADULTS)

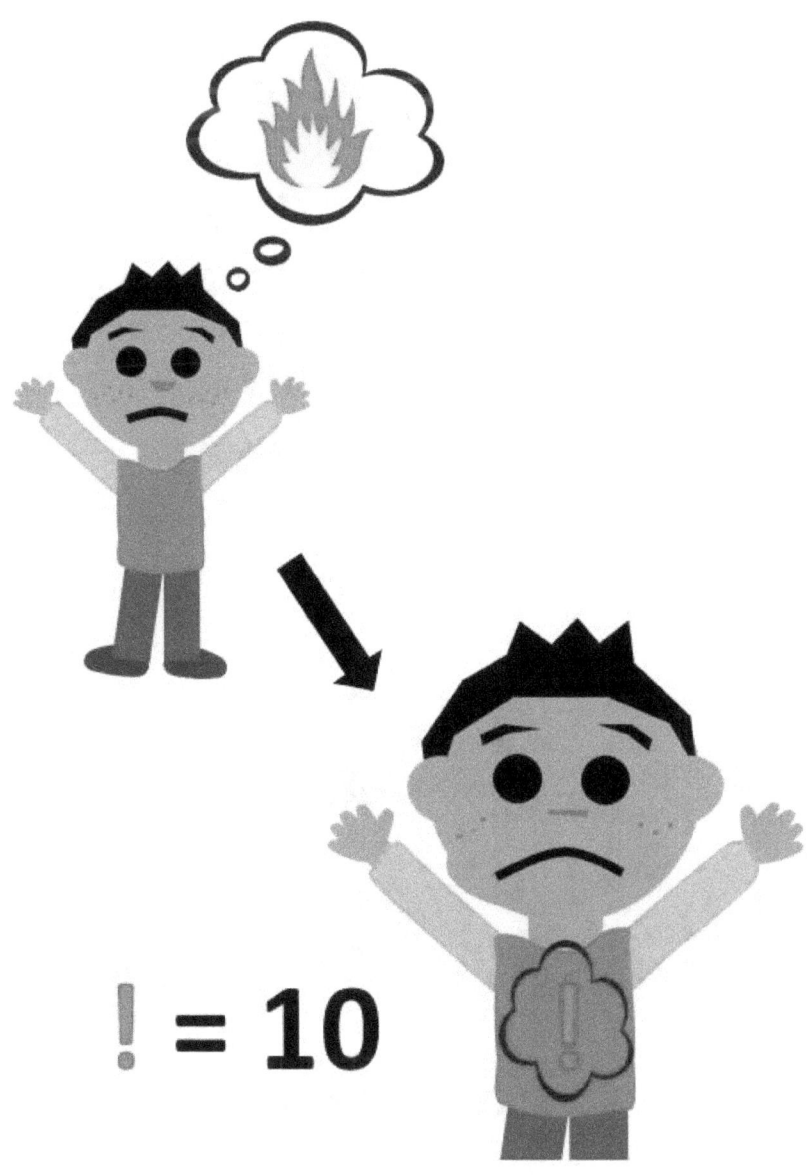

STEP 3 – FOLLOW (ADULTS)

STEP 4 – FORGET (ADULTS)

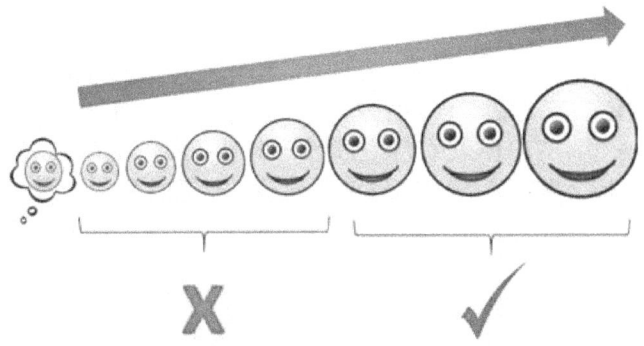

REPEAT FROM STEP 2 – FEEL (ADULTS)

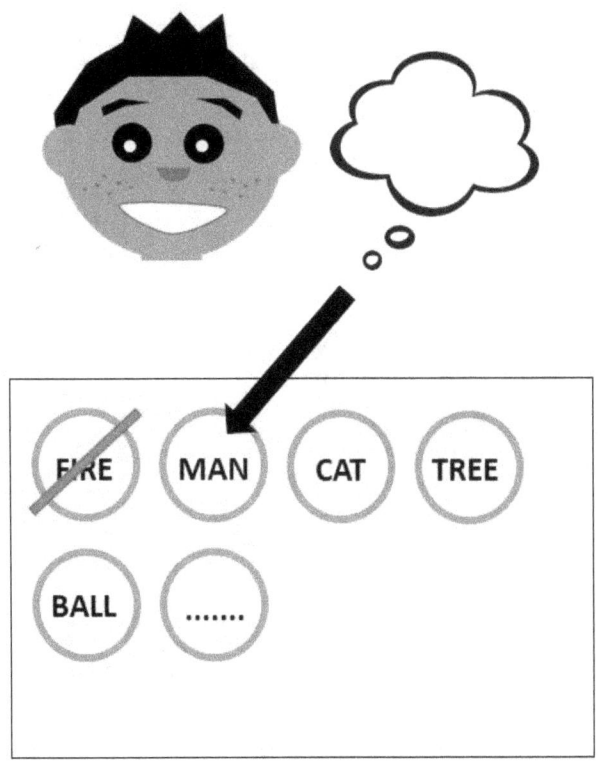

COMPLETE SCRIPT FOR ADULTS - STEP 1 – 'FIND'

TO HELP YOU RESOLVE THE FEELINGS AND THOUGHTS AND ANXIETY YOU'VE BEEN HAVING I'M JUST GOING TO TALK YOU THROUGH THIS SIMPLE GRAPH SO WE UNDERSTAND WHY WE HAVE BEEN FEELING THE WAY WE DO...

AND THIS GRAPH IS THEN GOING TO LEAD US ON TO IDENTIFYING THE CAUSES AND THAT'S WHAT WE ARE THEN GOING TO USE THE EASY EMDR ON, TO RESOLVE THOSE FEELINGS AND MEMORIES.

(explain and talk through the anxiety graph – a copy of which can be found at Chapter 16.)

SO NOW WE KNOW WHAT CAUSES THE ANXIETY WE NOW HAVE TO FIGURE OUT EXACTLY WHAT ALL THESE BUILDING BLOCKS ARE.

AND WE ARE GOING TO DO THAT BY DRAWING AND LABELLING SOME CIRCLES NICE AND SIMPLY.

IT'S NOT A COMPETITION HOW MANY CIRCLES YOU DRAW, SOME PEOPLE DRAW ONLY ONE, OTHERS DRAW 4 CIRCLES, OR 10, 20, SOME PEOPLE DRAW 40 OR MORE IT DOESN'T MATTER.

EACH CIRCLE ACTS AS A LABEL FOR A DISTRESSING MEMORY. THAT'S ALL IT IS. THINK OF EACH CIRCLE AS A SNAPSHOT IMAGE, LIKE A POLAROID PHOTO THAT'S BEEN NAMED.

ALL WE ARE LOOKING FOR TO BE WRITTEN IN EACH CIRCLE IS JUST ONE OR TWO WORDS THAT LABEL OR NAME OR DESCRIBE THAT PHOTO, OR SNAPSHOT IMAGE, THAT MEMORY.

LET ME GIVE YOU AN EXAMPLE I'VE MADE UP:

A TRAUMATIC MEMORY I HAVE IS FALLING OUT OF A CHERRY TREE.

SO THE LABEL I'M GOING TO WRITE COULD BE 'TREE' OR 'CHERRY TREE' OR 'FALL' OR 'ACCIDENT' – AS LONG AS YOU KNOW WHAY THE WORD RELATES TO THAT'S ALL WE NEED.

IF YOU FEEL THE WORD COULD CAUSE EMBARRASSMENT OR YOU DON'T WANT TO DISCLOSE IT THAT'S PERFECTLY OK, INSTEAD YOU CAN ABBREVIATE IT OR CHOOSE A CODE WORD. LIKE 'A' 'B' 'C' OR ORANGE OR BANANNA.

THIS IS WHY EMDR IS NON VERBAL YOU NEVER NEED TO EXPLAIN OR DISCUSS OR ELABORATE ON WHAT THE MEANING OF THE WORD IS – IT'S CONFIDENTIAL TO YOU, WE ARE NOT GOING TO TALK OR DISCUSS WHAT YOU'VE WRITTEN OK.

SO TO BEGIN WE ARE JUST GOING TO START BY TAKING SOME DEEP BREATHS TO RELAX US A LITTLE, THIS HELPS WITH RECALING ALL THOSE MEMORIES WE'RE LOOKNG FOR.

CLOSE YOUR EYES.

BREATHE IN FOR 4 FILLING YOUR LUNGS AND SHOULDERS.

HOLD IT... HOLD IT…

BREATHE OUT SLOWLY FOR 8 EXHALE ALL THE AIR.

BREATHE IN FOR 4 FILLING YOUR LUNGS AND SHOULDERS.

HOLD IT... HOLD IT...

BREATHE OUT SLOWLY FOR 8 EXHALE ALL THE AIR

BREATHE IN FOR 4 FILLING YOUR LUNGS AND SHOULDERS.

HOLD IT... HOLD IT... HOLD IT...

BREATHE OUT SLOWLY FOR 8 EXHALE ALL THE AIR

OPEN YOUR EYES FEELING SO MUCH MORE RELAXED.

(Use a black or blue pen YOU draw a medium sized circle top left corner)

SO THERE'S OUR FIRST CIRCLE.

IN A MINUTE YOU ARE GOING TO WRITE JUST ONE OR TWO WORDS IN THAT CIRCLE.

WRITE THE NAME OR USE A CODE WORD OF A TRAUAMTIC MEMORY THOUGHT OR FEELING.

AS SOON AS YOU'VE WRITTEN IN THE CIRCLE DRAW ANOTHER CIRCLE THE SAME SIZE TO THE RIGHT OF THE FIRST CIRCLE.

FOCUS ON THE BLANK CIRCLE YOU'VE JUST DRAWN, BY DOING THIS YOU WON'T FOCUS ON WHAT YOU'VE JUST WRITTEN.

JUST WRITE ONE OR TWO WORDS IN THAT CIRCLE OF ANOTHER TRAUMATIC MEMORY, THOUGHT OR FEELING, JUST WRITE WHAT COMES INTO YOUR MIND.

DRAW ANOTHER CIRCLE AND WRITE WHAT COMES INTO YOUR MIND.

DRAW ANOTHER CIRCLE AND WRITE WHAT COMES INTO YOUR MIND.

(if the subject doesn't draw a circle simply ask them quietly to DRAW A CIRCLE and point to the place where the circle should be drawn, remind them to FOCUS ON THE BLANK CIRCLE they have just drawn)

(let them continue until they become stuck or have finished)

(if they are STUCK and they will say this or just not write anything)

IF YOU FEEL STUCK JUST CLOSE YOUR EYES.

BREATHE IN FILLING YOUR LUNGS AND SHOULDERS.

HOLD IT... HOLD IT...

BREATHE OUT SLOWLY EXHALE ALL THE AIR.

BREATHE IN FILLING YOUR LUNGS AND SHOULDERS.

HOLD IT... HOLD IT...

BREATHE OUT SLOWLY EXHALE ALL THE AIR.

BREATHE IN FILLING YOUR LUNGS AND SHOULDERS.

HOLD IT... HOLD IT... HOLD IT...

BREATHE OUT SLOWLY EXHALE ALL THE AIR.

KEEP YOUR EYES CLOSED AND CONTINUE TO BREATHE NORMALY, IN A MOMENT OPEN YOUR EYES, FOCUS ON THE CIRCLE YOU'VE JUST DRAWN AND WRITE WHAT COMES INTO YOUR MIND.

OPEN YOUR EYES AND WRITE WHAT COMES INTO YOUR MIND.

(the subject will start to write again and the process continues, if they become stuck again simply ask the subject to close their eyes and instruct them in the breathing exercise all over again)

(at some point the subject will just stop and they will categorically KNOW they have finished, it's a very different feeling and body language to someone who is 'stuck')

(once they have finished you can move onto the next step, but only after you've checked everything you need to cover is recorded in one of the circles drawn)

AS YOU NOW LOOK OVER EVERYTHING THAT YOU'VE REMEMBERED IS THERE ANYTHING YOU CAN REMEMBER THAT YOU'VE LEFT OUT, IS THERE ANYTHING ELSE YOU'D LIKE TO ADD OR WORK ON?

(that question will lead to two answers; NO or YES, and if it's a YES simply ask the subject to draw another circle and label that memory, remember to ask the same question again! Don't assume there was only one memory left out)

(what we have covered here is an INDIRECT approach, if you are concerned they haven't addressed the issues you are aware of change the approach to become DIRECTED)

IS THE ISSUE YOU MENTIONED RECORDED HERE?

(again the subject will answer YES and probably show you but if NO, just ask them to draw a circle and label that memory)

(if they chose not to you must respect that decision and do not push the subject, perhaps come back to the therapy when they feel more comfortable)

YOU'VE DONE REALLY WELL!

(move straight on avoid discussing what has been written)

NOW WE NEED TO GRADE THEM, FOR THIS WE USE A RED PEN.

NOW GRADE THE MEMORIES BY WRITING A NUMBER IN EACH CIRCLE FROM 0 – 10. FEEL THE NUMBER DON'T THINK OF IT.

YOUR MIND WILL INTUITIVELY KNOW WHAT THE NUMBER IS. 0 IS THE LOWEST AND 10 BEING 10 THE HIGHEST.

THIS NUMBER REPRESENTS HOW 'BOTHERED' YOU ARE BY WHAT'S WRITTEN IN THE CIRCLE, OR HOW PAINFUL IT FEELS, OR HOW DISTRESSING THE MEMORY IS WHEN YOU THINK ABOUT IT.

WRITE THE NUMBER IN EACH CIRCLE IN RED, THEN MOVE STRAIGHT ONTO THE NEXT CIRCLE AND JUST KEEP GOING THERE'S NO NEED TO DWELL, JUST WRITE THE NUMBER THAT COMES INTO YOUR MIND.

(as they go along add up the numbers, they will give you a total)

(once you have the total you can refer them back to the Anxiety Graph and point to them where they now sit on that chart)

(it's at this stage for the first time they actually realise why they feel the way they feel, because they can see it on the graph)

SO THIS IS WHY YOU FEEL THE WAY YOU DO BECAUSE OF THE ACCUMULATIVE EFFECT OF THE TRAUMAS YOU'VE GONE THROUGH WHICH ADDS UP TO .... (say the total number) WHICH RELATES TO HOW STRESSED OR ANXIOUS YOU FEEL.

A SCORE BETWEEN 0-25 MEANS YOU WONT FEEL ANYTHING.

A SCORE BETWEEN 25-50 MEANS YOU WILL FEEL STRESSED.

A SCORE BETWEEN 50-75 MEANS YOU WILL BE EXPERIENCING ANXIETY IN YOUR DAILY LIFE AND YOUR BEHAVIOUR WILL START TO CHANGE AS YOUR MIND STARTS TO DISTRACT ITSELF FROM THE ANXIETY ITS FEELING.

AND OVER 75 IS WHERE WE PERHAPS START TO SEE REAL PHYSICAL CHANGES IN THE BODY AND YOU MAY EVEN FEEL SUICIDAL.

NOW YOU'VE SEEN THAT PROBABLY FOR THE FIRST TIME EVER, DOES THAT MAKE SENSE AS TO WHY YOU ARE FEELING THE WAY YOU ARE?

SO NOW WE'RE GOING TO WORK OUT WHICH MEMORIES WE ACTUALLY NEED TO WORK ON AND WHICH ONES WE CAN CROSS OFF.

WE CAN NOW DELETE ANY MEMORY GRADED 4 OR LOWER, ONLY IF YOU FEEL IT'S OK TO REMOVE IT.

(any memory graded 4 is border line, some memories can be deleted, others should stay and be worked on, it's the subject's choice)

IF YOU FEEL IT SHOULD STAY THEN JUST LET ME KNOW AND WE CAN LEAVE IT TO WORK ON.

ONCE THE HIGHER GRADED MEMORIES HAVE BEEN REPROCESSED YOUR MIND WILL USUALLY START TO THEN PROCESS THESE LOWER GRADE TRAUMAS ON THEIR OWN.

SO YOU SEE WE DON'T NEED TO TREAT EVERY MEMORY YOU'VE EVER HAD.

(but before you do always ask permission before crossing any one out – find the memories 4 and under and ask if you can delete each one then put a line through each one)

IS IT OK TO CROSS OUT THIS ONE?

(if they are unsure KEEP the circle)

AND THIS ONE?

(if there are no memories 4 or under then just jump to 'moving on'*)

WELL DONE THAT'S A GREAT START!

BY DELETING THESE WE'VE NOW ALREADY REDUCED THE NUMBER OF MEMORIES WE NEED TO TREAT SPEEDING UP YOUR TREATMENT.

*MOVING ON – WE'RE NOW GOING TO SPEED UP THE PROCESS SAFELY AGAIN BY GROUPING THE REMAINING MEMORIES WHERE POSSIBLE.

ARE ANY OF THESE MEMORIES CONNECTED, HAVE ANY OF THE MEMORIES HERE HAPPENED AT THE SAME TIME, IF SO CAN THEY BE GROUPED?

POINT OUT THE ONES THAT ARE GROUPED, AND I'LL DRAW A LINE CONNECTNG THEM.

THERE'S NO NEED TO EXPLAIN TO ME WHY.

(now draw a line between each circle joining them together, there maybe 3-10 circles grouped, just draw a line between each one, if lines start to cross draw two very small straight lines like a bridge or bracket recording the direction of flow)

GREAT NOW WE'VE GROUPED ALL THOSE WE CAN WORK ON THEM AS A GROUP AT THE SAME TIME, SO NOW WE HAVE (count the number of groups and single memories on the paper) .... AREAS OF TRAUMA TO TREAT RATHER THAN .... (say the total starting number before deletion and grouping).

YOU CAN SEE HOW GROUPING MEMORIES SPEEDS UP THE TREATMENT PROCESS.

WE'RE NOW GOING TO MOVE ONTO THE ACTUAL EMDR.

MOVE ONTO STEP 2 'FEEL' – FOR ADULTS

OK WE ARE NOW GOING TO WORK ON THE FIRST MEMORY SO JUST CLOSE YOUR EYES.

(use the breathing technique 4 in 8 out, to relax the subject)

BREATHE IN FILLING YOUR LUNGS AND SHOULDERS.

HOLD IT... HOLD IT...

BREATHE OUT SLOWLY EXHALE ALL THE AIR.

BREATHE IN FILLING YOUR LUNGS AND SHOULDERS.

HOLD IT... HOLD IT...

BREATHE OUT SLOWLY EXHALE ALL THE AIR.

BREATHE IN FILLING YOUR LUNGS AND SHOULDERS.

HOLD IT... HOLD IT... HOLD IT...

BREATHE OUT SLOWLY EXHALE ALL THE AIR.

I'M NOW GOING TO SAY A WORD TO YOU, AND WHEN I DO JUST ALLOW YOUR MIND TO GO ALL THE WAY BACK IN TIME TO AN EARLIER MEMORY CONNECTED WITH WHATEVER THE WORD ....(insert word from circle)........ MEANS TO YOU.

(use the words as written in the circle you are working on)

(repeat)

JUST ALLOW YOUR MIND TO GO BACK IN TIME TO AN EARLIER MEMORY CONNECTED WITH WHATEVER THE WORD/S .... MEANS TO YOU.

(repeat again the words)

JUST TELL ME WHEN YOU'RE THERE, WHEN YOU'RE IN THAT MEMORY.

(they will either say "I'm there" or nod their head)

WHERE CAN YOU *FEEL* THAT IN YOUR BODY?

(emphasise *FEEL*)

(they will either tell you or point to an area in their body)

HOW BAD IS THAT FEELING ON A SCALE OF 0-10?

(as soon as the subject grades the feeling immediately compare the RED number written in the MEMORY MAP)

(they should be the same or within 3 points higher or lower – if so move onto the next phase - FOLLOW which is the EMDR treatment)

(or if the memory isn't causing any feeling in the body then that memory isn't the cause of the anxiety - move onto the VISUALISATION TECHNIQUE below which starts IMAGINE A SCREEN....)

(if the numbers are very different this is an indicator that the subjects mind is not fully engaged – use the script below to deepen the engagement in the memory - ensure your subject's eyes are still closed)

KEEP YOUR EYES CLOSED.

IMAGINE A SCREEN JUST IN FRONT OF YOUR MIND.

NOW PROJECT AN IMAGE OF THE MEMORY ONTO THE SCREEN IT CAN BE A STILL IMAGE OR A MOVING IMAGE.

NOW REACH OUT WITH YOUR MIND AND FIND THE DIAL MARKED COLOUR AND TURN THE COLOUR OF THE IMAGE UP.

MAKE THE IMAGE BRIGHTER AND CLEARER AS IF YOU ARE ACTUALLY THERE.

(wait 10 seconds)

NOW REACH OUT WITH YOUR MIND AND FIND THE DIAL MARKED VOLUME AND TURN THE SOUND OF THE IMAGE UP.

MAKE THE IMAGE LOUDER AND CLEARER AS IF YOU ARE ACTUALLY THERE SO YOU CAN HEAR ABSOLUTELY EVERYTHING.

(wait 10 seconds)

WHERE CAN YOU FEEL THAT IN YOUR BODY NOW?

(emphasise the word NOW)

HOW BAD IS THAT FEELING ON A SCALE OF 0-10?

(the number should now be similar to the original MEMORY MAP)

(you can now move onto the EMDR Treatment, which will REDUCE this feeling and TURN DOWN or DESENSITISE the subject to the memory)

"KEEP YOUR EYES CLOSED"

MOVE ONTO STEP 3 'FOLLOW' – FOR ADULTS

(hold up your left hand to emphasise keeping their head straight, hold up your right hand and move your fingers into position ready)

OPEN YOUR EYES, KEEP YOUR HEAD STILL – AND FOLLOW MY FINGERS LEFT AND RIGHT (move fingers left and right - ensure eyes track and follow fully left and right)

KEEP FOLLOWING MY FINGERS, KEEP YOUR HEAD PERFECTLY STILL.

(you may have to repeat this at any time and more than once as they may easily forget as the process continues)

KEEP FOCUSSING ON THAT OLD MEMORY AND THAT OLD FEELING AS IT STARTS TO COME ALL THE WAY DOWN.

WHAT NUMBER WOULD YOU LIKE IT TO GO DOWN TO? A ZERO... A ONE... OR A TWO?

KEEP FOCUSSING ON THAT OLD MEMORY AND THAT OLD FEELING AS IT STARTS TO COME ALL THE WAY DOWN.

THE MORE IT COMES DOWN THE CALMER YOU FEEL, THE CALMER YOU FEEL THE MORE IT COMES DOWN AS YOUR MIND KNOWS EXACTLY WHAT IT NEEDS TO FIND TO HEAL RIGHT NOW DOESN'T IT.

(keep moving fingers with eyes following for approx. 10 seconds or if the eyes blink this is a good indicator the number has gone down so ask again...)

KEEP FOCUSING ON THAT OLD MEMORY AND THAT OLD FEELING - WHAT NUMBER HAS IT COME DOWN TO NOW?

(ensure they respond with a number, the method is to just keep going moving your fingers with eyes following until that number comes all the way down to the required number)

KEEP FOCUSING ON THAT OLD MEMORY AND THAT OLD FEELING - WHAT NUMBER HAS IT COME DOWN TO NOW?

(it will decrease number by number or it may drop or decrease in 2's, 3's, 4's or drop even more rapidly)

HUM HUM...

HUM HUM...

HUM HUM...

(keep acknowledging without words that you're still paying attention)

(when they get close to the desired number say...)

AND FINALLY....... LET GO! WHAT'S IT COME DOWN TO NOW?

(STOP when they say TWO, ONE or ZERO whatever number they choose)

CLOSE YOUR EYES.

MOVE ONTO STEP 4 'FORGET' – FOR ADULTS

OPEN YOUR EYES.

(ask 2 or 3 questions to confuse from the list below or make up your own)

LIST THE COLOURS OF THE RAINBOW IN ALPHABETICAL ORDER – GO!
WHAT'S THE OPPOSITE OF PURPLE?
WHAT IS PAPER MADE FROM?
WHAT'S THE FOURTH PLANET FROM THE MOON?
SPELL BALLERINA WITH NO VOWELS?
WHAT'S THE HEAVIEST ANIMAL IN THE WORLD?
WHAT'S THE HIGHEST MOUNTAIN IN THE WORLD?
WHAT'S THE SMALLEST MOUNTAIN IN THE WORLD?
WHAT WAS YOUR BUDGIES NAME AGAIN?
WHAT'S THE FASTEST TRAIN IN THE WORLD?
WHAT'S THE SLOWEST TRAIN IN THE WORLD?
GIVE ME YOUR MOBILE TELEPHONE NUMBER BACKWARDS?
GIVE ME YOUR CAR REGISTRATION BACKWARDS?
WHAT IS THE CHEMICAL SYMBOL FOR GOLD?

WHAT IS WATER MADE UP OF?
HOW MANY FATHOMS IN A MILE?
WHAT'S THE LARGEST ANIMAL IN THE WORLD?
SPELL PSEUDONYM?
WHAT IS GLASS MADE FROM?
NAME THREE FLOWERS THAT ARE YELLOW?
NAME A FLOWER THAT'S GREEN?

(as soon as they are confused or you've asked 3 questions...)

CLOSE YOUR EYES.

GO BACK TO THE **OLD** MEMORY AND FOCUS ON THAT **OLD** FEELING AND TELL ME IF THE OLD **FEELING** IS STILL THERE, HAS IT GONE, OR IS IT THERE JUST A LITTLE BIT?

(if the feeling is still there JUST A LITTLE BIT then ask them...)

WHAT IS JUST A LITTLE BIT ON THE SCALE OF 0-10?"

(if it's a 1 or a 2 ask them....)

ARE YOU ARE OK WITH THAT?

(if YES stop and jump ahead to Evaluating Success on the next page, if NOT follow the steps below)

(or if it's a ZERO jump ahead to Evaluating Success on the next page)

(or)

(if it's a 3 or higher follow the steps below and ask the subject...)

WHERE CAN YOU FEEL IT IN YOUR BODY?

(wait for the reply)

HOW MUCH ON A SCALE OF 0-10?

(wait for the reply and hold up your fingers ready to restart again)

OPEN YOUR EYES.

(begin the Step three 'FOLLOW' EASY EMDR process again, it will go down again, Break State using different questions as above, ask them to refocus on the old memory and the old feeling and the feeling this time may have finally gone! Or if it's there just a bit again then start the process again)

(keep chipping away at the feeling, bringing the sensitivity down and rechecking and chip away a bit more etc. until its finally gone)

(evaluating the success)

NOW THAT THE FEELING HAS GONE / OR HAS COME DOWN TO THE LOW NUMBER YOU CHOSE, HOW GOOD DOES THAT NOW FEEL ON A NEW SCALE OF ONE TO SEVEN, ONE BEING OK, SEVEN BEING FANTASTIC!?

(wait for the answer - success should be 5, 6 or 7 - if it's 5 or higher congratulate them – and then why not ask them...)

HOW GOOD DO YOU NOW FEEL?

(but if it's a number 4 or lower this indicates trauma may not be resolved)

(so then ask the subject)

WHY DO YOU FEEL IT HASN'T BEEN RESOLVED, WHY DOESN'T IT FEEL THAT GOOD?

(wait for the reply)

OK SO NOW WRITE ONE WORD DESCRIBING THIS IN A NEW CIRCLE ON YOUR EXISTING MEMORY MAP.

(work on this now and jump back to Step 2 'FEEL' and repeat until it is resolved, once this has been resolved then just go back to the Memory Map and start the whole process again)

Chapter 16

Conduct a Session for Older Children

SCRIPTS & ILLUSTRATIONS - OLDER CHILDREN

STEP 1 - FIND

STEP 2 – FEEL (OLDER CHILDREN)

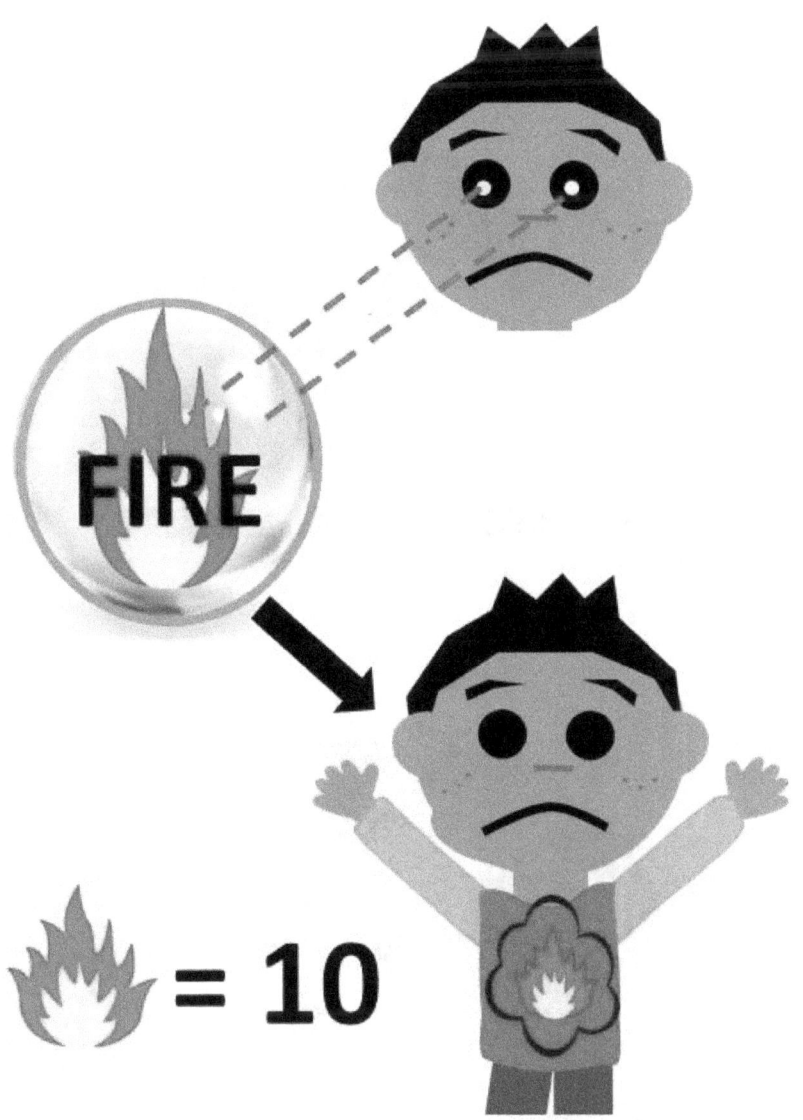

STEP 3 – FOLLOW (OLDER CHILDREN)

STEP 4 – FORGET (OLDER CHILDREN)

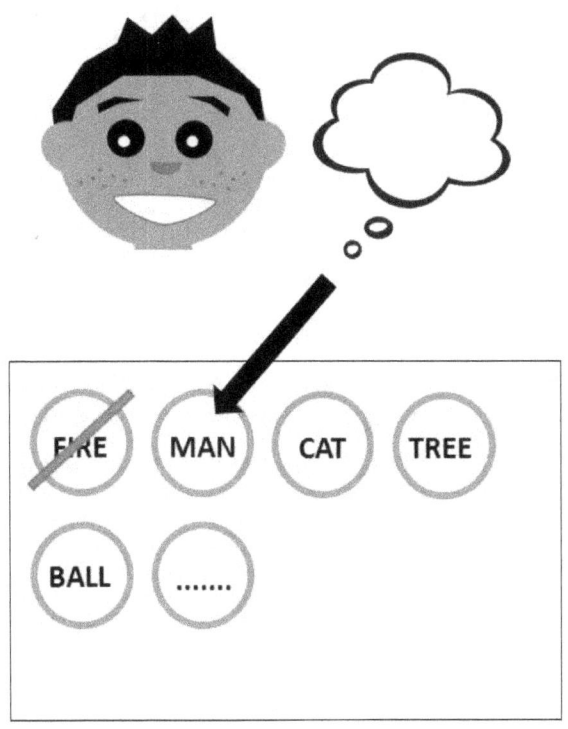

COMPLETE SCRIPT OLDER CHILDREN

STEP 1 – 'FIND'

(explain the fireworks story)

SOMETIMES WHEN WE FIX THE SAD MEMORIES IN OUR HEAD IT CAN BE LIKE A FIREWORK GOING OFF!

SOMETIMES THEY JUST SPARKLE WITH A LITTLE BANG, SOMETIMES THEY GO OFF WITH A BIG BANG! BUT SOON AS THEY DO THEY ALL START TO FIZZLE OUT AND DISAPPEAR.

ONCE A FIREWORK HAS BEEN LIT AND HAS GONE OFF IT CAN NEVER BE RE-LIT AGAIN CAN IT – IT'S FINISHED! IT'S GONE!

SO IF WE FIND ONES WITH BIG BANGS AND WE GET A BIT SCARED DON'T WORRY THEY'RE NOT REAL AND WILL FIZZLE OUT.

AND WE CAN ALWAYS GO TO A SAFE NICE PLACE – I'LL SHOW YOU HOW:

CAN YOU THINK OF A SAFE NICE PLACE RIGHT NOW? WHERE WOULD YOU LIKE TO GO TO FEEL SAFE? HOW ABOUT YOUR HOME, BEDROOM, ON HOLIDAY OR A NICE BEACH!

(remember a child's home or bedroom may not be safe for a child so expect anything to come up and if so ask them to create a magical space in their mind. Once they have named this place ask them to close their eyes)

THAT'S A NICE PLACE, NOW CLOSE YOUR EYES AND IMAGINE BEING THERE.

CAN YOU TELL ME ALL ABOUT WHERE YOU ARE? WHAT COLOURS AND THINGS CAN YOU SEE? HOW DO YOU FEEL?

(once you know they feel safe go on to explain)

NOW YOU CAN GO BACK TO THIS PLACE WHENEVER I ASK YOU TO AND YOU WILL BE SAFE – LETS TRY IT NOW.

WHAT DID YOU DO YESTERDAY?

(after a little while ask them firmly)

CLOSE YOUR EYES AND GO TO YOUR SAFE PLACE NOW! CAN YOU DESCRIBE IT AGAIN TO ME - AND HOW DO YOU NOW FEEL?

(it will be the same as before and you can now proceed safely)

(remember: if during the MEMORY MAPPING process they become distressed enough that they cannot continue you MUST take control of the situation and instruct them firmly to listen to your voice)

CLOSE YOUR EYES AND GO TO YOUR SAFE PLACE NOW!

DESCRIBE IT TO ME TELL ME WHERE YOU ARE AND HOW YOU FEEL.

(your subject will begin to calm, now use the 4 IN 8 OUT breathing technique you have already learnt and practiced this will reduce the anxiety)

(it is important to only intervene where absolutely necessary)

(it is helpful to first explain to the older child what we are trying to achieve, drawing the Anxiety Graph may probably be of benefit)

(if treating 'older children' then educating them about how anxiety builds from a young age will be life changing for them, so if you feel its age appropriate then DO use this graph or both systems together)

(do that now if appropriate)

TO HELP YOU RESOLVE THE FEELINGS AND THOUGHTS AND ANXIETY YOU'VE BEEN HAVING I'M JUST GOING TO TALK YOU THROUGH THIS SIMPLE GRAPH SO WE UNDERSTAND WHY YOU'VE BEEN FEELING THE WAY YOU DO.

THIS GRAPH IS THEN GOING TO HELP US IDENTIFY THE CAUSES AND THAT'S WHAT WE ARE THEN GOING TO USE THE EMDR ON, TO RESOLVE THOSE FEELINGS AND MEMORIES.

(explain and talk through the Anxiety Graph – a copy of which can be found at Chapter 16.)

(but if this explanation is not age appropriate miss out the graph completely and perhaps use the explanation script below to teach a child what anxiety is WITHOUT the graph)

THOSE FEELINGS AND MEMORIES CAN FEEL LIKE BEING UNDER A SPELL WHICH MAKES CHILDREN DO THINGS THEY WOULDN'T NORMALLY DO AND CHANGE THIER BEHAVIOUR

AS WE KNOW THERE ARE GOOD SPELLS AND SAD SPELLS, THE SAD SPELLS MAKE US FEEL UNWELL, THE GOOD SPELLS HELP US GET WELL.

WHAT WE ARE GOING TO DO NOW IS USE THE GOOD SPELLS TO MAKE US FEEL SO MUCH BETTER.

NOW TO BE ABLE TO DO MAGIC WE NEED A WAND, HERE WE ARE!

AND WE CAN USE A CRYSTAL BALL (if you don't have one just draw a circle to represent the crystal ball) SOME MAGIC PAPER AND A PEN AND A MAGICAL 'MEMORY FLASK', TO CONTAIN THE MEMORIES IN.

(show the child all these items and let them explore them)

MEMORY FLASKS HAVE BEEN USED THROUGHOUT MAGICAL HISTORY TO HOLD THINGS LIKE:

GENIES, POTIONS, SPELLS AND MEMORIES.

WHAT WE ARE GOING TO DO IS USE THE MAGIC WAND TO FIND OUR SAD MEMORIES AND EXTRACT THEM WITH THE WAND FROM OUR HEAD AND PUT THE CHOSEN MEMORY INSIDE THE BOTTLE.

THEN WE ARE GOING TO GIVE THE MEMORY A NAME AND LABEL THE BOTTLE.

TO BE ABLE TO LOOK AT THE MEMORY WE USE AN OLD MAGICAL DEVICE A 'CRYSTAL BALL' WHICH IS LIKE A MAGIC CIRCLE, WHICH WE USE TO PLACE THE MEMORY INTO.

AND THERE IT SWIRLS AROUND SO WE WILL BE ABLE TO SEE THE MEMORY.

AND THEN THAT'S IT DA DAH WE'VE FOUND THE MEMORY USING MAGIC.

LET'S HAVE A GO.

(you can show the child the illustrations of what you're about to do to make it easy to explain and understand and then show the child on yourself first)

OK SO I TAKE HOLD OF THE WAND

I PUT IT TO MY HEAD AND NOW I THINK OF THE SAD MEMORY

HMMM THERE IT IS!

NOW I SLOWLY PULL OUT THE MEMORY LIKE A BUBBLE AND AS IT STICKS TO THE END OF THE WAND I POP IT INTO THE MEMORY FLASK!

(describe the memory bubble being pulled out, describe the bubble appearing and comment on how you can see it and inform the child they can see it too as you place it into the flask. The child will inevitably agree. They are now 'engaged' in the process)

OK NOW YOU TRY! BUT BEFORE THAT WE ARE GOING TO ENTER A MAGICAL SPACE NICE AND CALMLY TOGETHER.

CLOSE YOUR EYES.

NOW BREATHE IN FILLING YOUR BODY UP WITH AIR.

HOLD IT... HOLD IT...

AND BREATHE OUT SLOWLY KEEP YOUR EYES CLOSED.

BREATHE IN AGAIN THAT'S RIGHT ALL THE WAY IN.

HOLD IT... HOLD IT...

AND BREATHE OUT ALL THE AIR SLOWLY.

AND ONE MORE TIME BREATHE ALL THE WAY IN...

HOLD IT... HOLD IT... HOLD IT...

AND BREATHE OUT SLOWLY.

AND OPEN YOUR EYES FEELING NICE AND CALM.

NOW PLACE THE WAND ON THE SIDE OF YOUR HEAD.

THAT'S RIGHT AND THINK OF THE MEMORY THAT YOU WOULD LIKE TO REMOVE.

ONCE YOU'VE THOUGHT OF THE MEMORY, YOU'RE NOW GOING TO PULL THE MEMORY OUT IN A BUBBLE BY USING THE WAND.

IMAGINE IT APPEARING AS YOU'VE SEEN IN THE PICTURES JUST AS I DID.

(if they choose not to see the bubble they are not engaged in the process and you should then ask the child why they cannot see the memory. It is important to go back and explain to them in order for them to feel better you are going to help them by removing the memory from their mind and giving the child the choice to let it go away using the wand)

(once they agree continue again placing the wand at the child's temple)

OK SO NOW PULL THE MEMORY OUT, THAT'S RIGHT THERE IT IS! AND THERE'S THE MEMORY BUBBLE ATTACHED TO THE WAND.

(make sure you have your Memory Flask to hand, or the empty jar or bottle with a lid ensuring there is NO label on the flask)

NOW WE PUT THE MEMORY INTO THE MAGICAL FLASK THAT WILL SAFELY STORE THE MEMORY WHERE YOU CAN STILL SEE IT – THAT'S RIGHT IN IT GOES!

(ensure the flask is always seen by the child and they do not look away)

AND THERE IS YOUR MEMORY SWIRLING ALL AROUND.

(acting surprised and excited)

AH THERE'S NO LABEL! OH NO!

SO HOW DO WE KNOW WHAT THIS MEMORY IS CALLED?

I KNOW! WE CAN GIVE THE MEMORY A LABEL, A NAME CANT WE.

OK HOW ABOUT YOU JUST GIVE ME ONE OR TWO WORDS TO DESCRIBE WHAT YOU'D LIKE TO CALL IT?

THAT'S REALLY GOOD WELL DONE!

NOW YOU SEE THE TOP OF THE BOTTLE WHAT SHAPE IS IT?

(turn the bottle to face the child so they can see the round top or opening)

A CIRCLE THAT'S RIGHT, SO LET'S DRAW THE TOP OF THE BOTTLE ON THE PAPER - THERE WE GO A CIRCLE! THAT'S THE TOP OF OUR BOTTLE, AND WE CAN WRITE THE NAME .... ON THE BOTTLE OR IN THE CIRCLE.

(write the label the child has given you in the circle - you have now written in the circle as if using the ADULT protocol)

SO LETS DRAW ANOTHER CIRCLE, ANOTHER BOTTLE AND NOW LETS FIND ANOTHER MEMORY AND PULL IT OUT AND PUT IT IN THE NEW BOTTLE JUST AS WE DID BEFORE – YOU CAN DRAW THE CIRCLES NOW.

(repeat the wand memory extraction process again)

NOW TAKE THE WAND AGAIN

THIS TIME YOU CAN TAKE THE MEMORY AND PUT INTO DIRECTLY INTO THE TOP OF THE FLASK WE'VE DRAWN

AND WRITE THE NAME OF THE MEMORY IN THAT CIRCLE – THAT'S RIGHT!

(you now have the second memory recorded but you've speeded up the process by cutting out the use of the flask. You can put this to one side now as we are just going to use the circles)

NOW FOR THE THIRD MEMORY HOW ABOUT WE JUST USE THE PEN AS IF IT WAS A WAND! DRAW THE NEXT CIRCLE TO GET THE FLASK READY FOR THE NEXT MEMORY – THAT'S RIGHT.

(you can buy a pen that looks like a wand if this helps)

NOW USE THE PEN AS YOUR WAND TO PULL OUT THE NEXT MEMORY, PLACE THE MEMORY INTO THE NEXT CIRCLE, AND WRITE IN THE CIRCLE THE NAME FOR THIS MEMORY.

(just keep going until the child is finished - if the child is stuck simply follow the same adult protocol for being 'stuck' by closing eyes and taking three breaths in and out)

(what we have covered here is an INDIRECT approach if you are concerned they haven't addressed the issues you discussed, then you can change the approach to become DIRECTED - simply ask them directly)

IS THE ISSUE OF .... (name the subject matter) WE DISCUSSED HERE ON THE PAPER SOMEWHERE?

(they may answer YES and show you but if it's a NO ask them to draw a circle and label that memory)

(if they chose not to you must respect that decision)

(do not push the subject or they will simply not engage in the process, perhaps come back to the therapy when they feel more comfortable)

(once you have all the circles completed you will now be able to move onto grading the memories on the scale of BEING BOTHERED before you move onto the actual EMDR, where you will use the Magic Circles drawn as a representation of the Crystal Ball)

(in order to grade the memories use a RED pen)

WELL DONE SO NOW WE ARE GOING TO GRADE THE MEMORIES BY WRITING A NUMBER IN EACH CIRCLE FROM 0 – 10.

YOU WILL KNOW WHAT THE NUMBER IS, IT'S THE FIRST NUMBER THAT COMES INTO YOUR HEAD.

0 IS LOW AND 10 IS HIGH. THIS NUMBER REPRESENTS HOW 'BOTHERED' YOU ARE BY THE MEMORY IN THE CIRCLE, ITS VERY EASY JUST LOOK AT THAT MEMORY AND WRITE THE NUMBER IN THE CIRCLE THERE.

WELL DONE! NOW KEEP GOING AND LETS GRADE THEM ALL.

(use the Bothered Scale illustration if needed on Page 108 Chapter 9)

(add up the numbers they will give you a total, once you have the total you can refer back to the Anxiety Graph to see where the child sits and if this is what you expected – explain this to them if using the adult script below)

SO THIS IS WHY YOU FEEL THE WAY THEY DO BECAUSE OF THE ACCUMULATIVE EFFECT OF THE TRAUMAS YOU'VE GONE THROUGH WHICH ADDS UP TO .... (say the total number)

THIS SCORE RELATES TO HOW STRESSED OR ANXIOUS YOU FEEL.

A SCORE BETWEEN 0-25 MEANS YOU WONT FEEL ANYTHING.

A SCORE BETWEEN 25-50 MEANS YOU WILL FEEL STRESSED.

A SCORE BETWEEN 50-75 MEANS YOU WILL BE EXPERIENCING ANXIETY IN YOUR DAILY LIFE AND YOUR BEHAVIOUR WILL START TO CHANGE AS YOUR MIND STARTS TO DISTRACT ITSELF FROM THE ANXIETY IT'S FEELING.

AND OVER 75 IS WHERE WE PERHAPS START TO SEE REAL PHYSICAL CHANGES IN THE BODY (only say if age appropriate) AND YOU MAY EVEN FEEL SUICIDAL.

NOW YOU'VE SEEN THAT PROBABLY FOR THE FIRST TIME EVER, DOES THAT MAKE SENSE AS TO WHY YOU ARE FEELING THE WAY YOU ARE?

(if you're not using the adult version of the anxiety graph and you've used the magical spells explanations then start again from here)

SO NOW WE'RE GOING TO WORK OUT WHICH MEMORIES WE NEED TO USE OUR MAGIC ON TO MAKE THEM DISAPPEAR AND WHICH ONES WE DON'T SO WE CAN CROSS THEM OFF.

WE CAN NOW DELETE ANY MEMORY GRADED 4 OR LOWER, ONLY IF YOU FEEL IT'S OK TO REMOVE IT.

(any memory graded a 4 is on the border line some memories can be deleted, perhaps others should stay and be worked on, it's the subject's choice)

IF YOU FEEL IT SHOULD STAY THEN JUST LET ME KNOW AND WE CAN LEAVE IT TO USE OUR MAGIC SPELLS ON

(find the memories 4 and under and ask if you can delete and put a line through each one)

IS IT OK TO CROSS OUT THIS ONE?

(if they are unsure KEEP the circle)

AND THIS ONE?

(if there are no memories 4 or under then just simply move on*)

WELL DONE THAT'S A GREAT START!

(only group children's memories if there are enough to warrant this part of the therapy i.e. perhaps a whole page or more than one page)

WE'RE NOW GOING TO MOVE ONTO THE MAGIC SPELL USING OUR WAND TO FORGET ALL THESE MEMORIES.

WELL DONE, YOU'VE DONE REALLY REALY WELL!

(praise the child and go to EMDR script for Older Children using Magic)

MOVE ONTO STEP 2 - 'FEEL' (older children)

OK WE ARE NOW GOING TO WORK ON THE FIRST MEMORY SO JUST CLOSE YOUR EYES.

(use the breathing technique 4 in 8 out, to relax the subject)

BREATHE IN FILLING YOUR LUNGS AND SHOULDERS.

HOLD IT... HOLD IT...

BREATHE OUT SLOWLY EXHALE ALL THE AIR.

BREATHE IN FILLING YOUR LUNGS AND SHOULDERS.

HOLD IT... HOLD IT...

BREATHE OUT SLOWLY EXHALE ALL THE AIR.

BREATHE IN FILLING YOUR LUNGS AND SHOULDERS.

HOLD IT... HOLD IT... HOLD IT...

BREATHE OUT SLOWLY EXHALE ALL THE AIR.

I'M NOW GOING TO SAY A WORD TO YOU, AND WHEN I DO JUST ALLOW YOUR MIND TO GO ALL THE WAY BACK IN TIME TO AN EARLIER MEMORY CONNECTED WITH WHATEVER THE WORD ....(insert word from circle)........ MEANS TO YOU.

(use the words as written in the circle you are working on)

(repeat)

JUST ALLOW YOUR MIND TO GO BACK IN TIME TO AN EARLIER MEMORY CONNECTED WITH WHATEVER THE WORD/S .... MEANS TO YOU.

(repeat again the words)

JUST TELL ME WHEN YOU'RE THERE, WHEN YOU'RE IN THAT MEMORY.

(they will either say "I'm there" or nod their head)

WHERE CAN YOU *FEEL* THAT IN YOUR BODY?

(emphasise *FEEL*)

(they will either tell you or point to an area in their body)

HOW BAD IS THAT FEELING ON A SCALE OF 0-10?

(as soon as the subject grades the feeling immediately compare the RED number written in the MEMORY MAP to the actual number that the subject is 'feeling')

(They should be the same or within 3 points higher or lower – if so move onto the next phase – 'FOLLOW' which is the EMDR treatment)

KEEP YOUR EYES CLOSED.

(or)

(if the memory isn't causing any feeling in the body then that memory isn't the cause of the anxiety - move onto the VISUALISATION TECHNIQUE below which starts IMAGINE A SCREEN....)

(if they are very different this is an indicator that the subjects mind is not fully engaged – use the script below to deepen the engagement in the memory, ensure your subject's eyes are still closed)

IMAGINE A SCREEN JUST IN FRONT OF YOUR MIND.

NOW PROJECT AN IMAGE OF THE MEMORY ONTO THE SCREEN IT CAN BE A STILL IMAGE OR A MOVING IMAGE.

NOW REACH OUT WITH YOUR MIND AND FIND THE DIAL MARKED COLOUR AND TURN THE COLOUR OF THE IMAGE UP.

MAKE THE IMAGE BRIGHTER AND CLEARER AS IF YOU ARE ACTUALLY THERE.

(wait 10 seconds)

NOW REACH OUT WITH YOUR MIND AND FIND THE DIAL MARKED VOLUME AND TURN THE SOUND OF THE IMAGE UP.

MAKE THE IMAGE LOUDER AND CLEARER AS IF YOU ARE ACTUALLY THERE SO YOU CAN HEAR ABSOLUTELY EVERYTHING.

(wait 10 seconds)

WHERE CAN YOU FEEL THAT IN YOUR BODY *NOW*?

(emphasise the word NOW)

HOW BAD IS THAT FEELING ON A SCALE OF 0-10?

(the number should now be similar to the original MEMORY MAP)

(you can now move onto the EMDR Treatment, which will REDUCE this feeling and TURN DOWN or DESENSITISE the subject to the memory)

KEEP YOUR EYES CLOSED.

MOVE ONTO STEP 3 – 'FOLLOW' (older children)

OPEN YOUR EYES, KEEP YOUR HEAD STILL – AND FOLLOW THE WAND LEFT AND RIGHT.

KEEP FOLLOWING THE WAND.

(you may have to say this more than once as they may easily forget)

KEEP FOCUSSING ON THAT OLD MEMORY AND THAT OLD FEELING AS IT STARTS TO COME ALL THE WAY DOWN.

WHAT NUMBER WOULD YOU LIKE IT TO GO DOWN TO? A ZERO, A ONE, OR A TWO?

KEEP FOCUSSING ON THAT OLD MEMORY AND THAT OLD FEELING AS IT STARTS TO COME ALL THE WAY DOWN.

THE MORE IT COMES DOWN THE CALMER YOU FEEL, THE CALMER YOU FEEL THE MORE IT COMES DOWN.

(keep moving wand with eyes following for approx. 10 seconds or if the eyes blink this is a good indicator the number has gone down so ask again...)

KEEP FOCUSING ON THAT OLD MEMORY AND THAT OLD FEELING - WHAT NUMBER HAS IT COME DOWN TO NOW?

(they will respond with a number, the method is to just keep going moving your wand with eyes following until that number comes all the way down to the required number)

KEEP FOCUSING ON THAT OLD MEMORY AND THAT OLD FEELING - WHAT NUMBER HAS IT COME DOWN TO NOW?

(it will decrease number by number or it may drop or decrease in 2's, 3's, 4's or drop even more rapidly)

HUM HUM, HUM HUM, HUM HUM

(keep acknowledging without words that you're still paying attention, when they get close to the desired number say...)

AND FINALLY....... LET GO! WHAT'S IT COME DOWN TO NOW?

(STOP when they say TWO, ONE or ZERO whatever number they choose)

CLOSE YOUR EYES.

MOVE ONTO STEP 4 – 'FORGET' (Older children)

OPEN YOUR EYES.

(ask 2 or 3 questions to confuse from the list below or make up your own)

WHAT COLOUR IS GREEN & BLUE MIXED TOGETHER?
WHAT IS AN APPLE CROSSED WITH AN ORANGE?
WHAT IS A BRIDGE OVER A RAILWAY CALLED?
HOW MANY SPOTS DOES A LADY BIRD HAVE?

(as soon as they are confused or you've asked 3 questions...)

CLOSE YOUR EYES.

GO BACK TO THE **OLD** MEMORY AND FOCUS ON THAT **OLD** FEELING AND TELL ME IF THE OLD **FEELING** IS STILL THERE, HAS IT GONE, OR IS IT THERE JUST A LITTLE BIT?

(if the feeling is still there *JUST A LITTLE BIT* then ask them...)

WHAT IS JUST A LITTLE BIT ON THE SCALE OF 0-10?"

(if it's a 1 or a 2 ask them...)

ARE YOU ARE OK WITH THAT?

(if YES stop and jump ahead to Evaluating Success below, if NOT follow the steps below)

(or)

(if it's a ZERO jump ahead to **Evaluating the Success** below)

(or)

(if it's a 3 or higher follow the steps below and ask the subject...)

WHERE CAN YOU FEEL IT IN YOUR BODY?

(wait for the reply)

HOW MUCH ON A SCALE OF 0-10?

(wait for the reply and hold up the wand or fingers ready to restart again from the Step three 'FOLLOW' EASY EMDR process)

OPEN YOUR EYES.

(begin again, it will go down again, ask Break State questions using different questions as above, ask them to refocus on the old memory and the old feeling and the feeling this time may have finally gone - or if it's there just a bit again, then start the process again)

(keep chipping away at the feeling, bringing the sensitivity down and rechecking and chip away a bit more etc. until its finally gone)

(evaluating the success)

NOW THAT THE FEELING HAS GONE / OR HAS COME DOWN TO THE LOW NUMBER YOU CHOSE, HOW GOOD DOES THAT NOW FEEL ON A NEW SCALE OF ONE TO SEVEN, ONE BEING OK, SEVEN BEING FANTASTIC!?

(wait for the answer - success should be 5, 6 or 7 - if it's 5 or higher congratulate them – so why not then ask them...)

HOW DO YOU NOW FEEL?

(if it's a number 4 or lower this indicates trauma may not be resolved)

(so ask the subject)

WHY DO YOU FEEL IT HASN'T BEEN RESOLVED OR WHY DOESN'T IT FEEL THAT GOOD?

(wait for the reply)

OK SO NOW WRITE ONE WORD DESCRIBING THIS IN A NEW CIRCLE ON YOUR EXISTING MEMORY MAP.

(work on this now and jump back to Step 2 'FEEL' and repeat until it is resolved and once this has been resolved then just go back to the Memory Map and start the whole process again)

Chapter 17

Conduct a Session for Younger Children

SCRIPTS & ILLUSTRATIONS - YOUNGER CHILDREN

STEP 1 – 'FIND' (younger child)

STEP 2 – 'FEEL' (younger child)

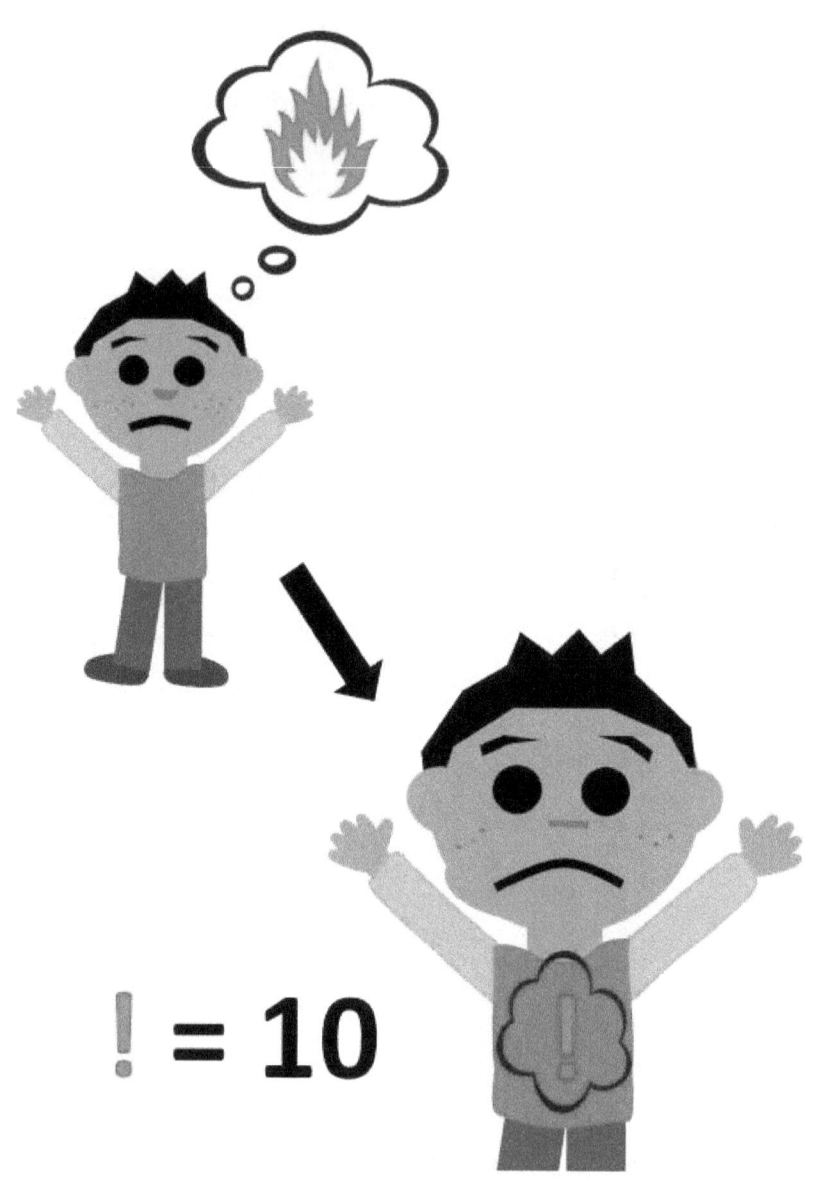

STEP 3 – 'FOLLOW' (younger child)

STEP 4 – 'FORGET' (younger child)

COMPLETE SCRIPT FOR YOUNGER CHILDREN
STEP 1 - 'FIND'

(as no detailed script is required for the step one for young children you can simply ask this question:)

DO YOU REMEMBER WHEN ....

(or)

SHALL WE HAVE A LOOK AT YOUR LOVELY PICTURE?

(use the Theraplay art work)

MOVE ONTO STEP 2 - 'FEEL' (younger child)

(as soon as they tell you what the memory is just ask the child...)

WHERE CAN YOU FEEL THAT INSIDE YOUR BODY?

(this step is very quick and easy as younger children don't over think this)

MOVE ONTO STEP 3 - 'FOLLOW' (younger child)

OPEN YOUR EYES.

AND NOW FOLLOW THE .... (use the name of the finger puppet dog, cat, mouse etc).

KEEP THINKING OF THAT MEMORY OF .... (name the memory they used).

KEEP FOLLOWING THE .... (finger puppet name).

IF YOU CAN STILL FEEL IT DON'T WORRY IT WILL START TO GO AWAY.

KEEP THINKING OF THAT MEMORY OF .... (name the memory they used).

KEEP FOLLOWING THE .... (finger puppet name).

IF YOU CAN STILL FEEL IT DON'T WORRY IT WILL KEEP GOING AWAY UNTIL IT'S......GONE!

JUST TELL ME WHEN IT'S GONE?

(at this stage the child may want to go off and play and that's ok)

(or if still engaged continue on)

MOVE ONTO STEP 4 - 'FORGET' (younger child)

OPEN YOUR EYES.

(break state by asking very simple questions such as:)

WHERE DO FISH LIVE?
WHAT NOISE DOES A FIRE ENGINE MAKE?
WHAT'S YOUR FAVOURITE SWEET?

(wait for the reply)

NOW TRY AND GO BACK TO THE OLD FEELING AND SEE IF IT'S THERE OR HAS IT GONE?

(wait for the reply - when feeling has finally 'GONE' remove finger puppet quickly and say...)

YES LOOK IT'S GONE!

WELL DONE! YOU'VE BEEN REALLY GOOD - SHALL WE GO AND PLAY NOW?

(if not gone completely or a 2 or higher then repeat eye tracking with the finger puppet)

(after a few days you can move onto the next memory and begin the entire process again allowing at least 2 days to pass)

Chapter 18

Ongoing Therapy – Mindfulness & MindMagic

The most helpful and simplest form of Therapy to follow EMDR is **MINDFULNESS**.

What is it?

Mindfulness is a simple mind & body therapy or process that helps people manage their thoughts and feelings and therefore improves over all mental health. It is widely used and recognised by all mental health organisations, hospitals and most charities and even schools. Importantly just like EMDR it is recommended by NICE "as a preventative practice for people with experience of recurrent depression", but has just like EMDR far wider applications.

Mindfulness exercises are ways of paying attention to the 'here and now' or the present moment, using techniques like meditation, breathing, and yoga. But contained here within this book EASY EMDR again has a very simple system that is proven to work without detailed training. It helps people to become more aware of their thoughts and feelings, so that instead of being overwhelmed by them, they can manage them or even simpler get rid of them so they do not become intrusive or effect daily life.

Mindfulness can be practiced on your own by children, young people and adults. There are different ways to practice mindfulness, group courses are often held and there are many online courses and mobile applications too where you can learn at home. It's important to understand you don't need to practice religion, be spiritual or even have a particular belief system to practice the EASY EMDR mindfulness technique. One of the best Apps is HEADSPACE which is highly recommended for further study. It's free to download and to use the initial courses. If you like it you can join but there's no obligation.

Why is MINDFULNESS beneficial after EMDR?

Mindfulness is a way of dealing with traumatic thoughts and daily thoughts non-judgmentally. Mindfulness is highly beneficial after EMDR because it allows the subject to continue the good positive work outside of the therapy session – so you don't need anyone else to help you maximise growth.

Mindfulness is actually already woven into the whole EMDR process, from focusing on the thoughts that are drawn into the circles, on focusing on our breath as we breathe in an out, on focusing on how our minds are adjusting to once traumatic thoughts and how our bodies' reaction to once traumatic thoughts have changed.

So it's no wonder it would be highly beneficial to practice easy mindfulness after EMDR, as you or your subject has already being doing it!

With its popularity in the East and West, research is widely reporting the positive effects of Mindfulness on the brain as it continues after EMDR to help reduce pain, anxiety and depression, whilst improving learning and even memory, which is often hit hardest during acute anxiety where loosing memory can be one of the first things to happen!

Practicing Mindfulness after EMDR is highly beneficial for people who have experienced trauma or stressful life events.

The combined approach of EMDR and Mindfulness helps people to continue to process residual final memories and also helps process new things that can be experienced in life.

Mindfulness is safe and can be carried out with the eyes closed or open, at home, at school where it is even now taught, in the office or even walking down the street. Mindfulness can be practiced in the shower, eating food, as a family or in a mini group session – basically everywhere outside of the therapy setting.

A main symptom of Stress, Trauma, Loss, PTSD, ADD, ADHD, Asperger, IBS, OCD, CPD, is anxiety as we now know. People use a variety of distraction behaviours to escape feeling the emotions, thoughts and feelings that remind them of the traumatic memories.

The survival strategy of distractions or addictions can make people feel disconnected from themselves, family, friends and in general the world they live in. Having PTSD or Post Traumatic Stress can also make it very difficult to concentrate on even the simplest of tasks. People can become withdrawn and feel very isolated from life.

These additional feelings can make it even harder for anyone to feel at ease in a mindful space. This is why it is recommended to practice Mindfulness AFTER EMDR and not before! It can simply be far too stressful and can retrigger even deeper emotions and responses.

How do I practice Mindfulness?

The best way to explain this is to give you a very simple exercise to perform as an adult, give this a try now and you'll see just how simple and effective the process is.

Difficulty: Easy

Time Required: 10 minutes

Find a comfortable position either lying on your back or sitting.

If you are sitting down, make sure that you keep your back straight and release the tension in your shoulders. Let them drop.

Close your eyes.

Focus your attention on your breathing. Simply pay attention to what it feels like in your body to slowly breathe in and out.

Now bring your attention to your stomach. Feel your stomach rise, expand and fall every time you breathe in and out.

Now focus your attention on the tip of your nose. Focus your closed eyes on the tip of your nose.

Anytime that you notice a thought comes into your mind no matter what that thought was, focus the energy at the tip of your nose and say in your mind JUST GO..... and imagine pushing that energy like a cone, smoke ring or donut from the tip of your nose outward and pushing that thought out of your mind. With a little practice you will see the thought just vanish. As you say JUST GO you can also breathe out calmly using your breath to push the thought away too with an Ohhhhhhhhhhh sound coming from the back of your throat.

If you mind's attention has wandered away from the tip of your nose then just refocus your attention here again. All our minds wander it's completely normal, so don't worry when it does, it will happen, just regain the focus on your nose.

The more you practice JUST GOooohhhhhhhhhh pushing the thoughts away, the longer the gap will be in between each new thought arriving, and as such we are learning to take back control and calm our mind simply and easily!

Continue as long as you would like but 10-15 mins is very beneficial, especially if you practice this daily! Just 10-15 mins a day for 7 days in a row will help calm your mind and you will notice the difference!

Calming the Mind

In the Far East calming the mind during meditation is often referred to as 'Taming your chattering monkey' which simply means learning to stop the constant barrage of thoughts that go round in our heads – which is often the case with people suffering from anxiety!

In the West it's also clinically referred to as 'rumination' where our minds chew and chew over events again and again in our mind - just like cows that chew & chew grass again and again to make milk. That process in cows is also called 'rumination' which is why cows are called 'ruminants'!

So if your mind is often bombarded with negative thoughts you can use this simple exercise or technique any time of the day anywhere to calm your mind and push those negative thoughts away. I still use this technique daily in my own life to great effect, as humans we are all susceptible to intrusive thoughts whether in bed at night, when waking up, or even just walking down the street or driving.

If you're driving you're NOT in a safe place to close your eyes, or even just walking it's NOT safe to close your eyes – but you don't need to! With THIS technique you can also just push those thoughts out of your mind by focusing on the thought, moving your attention to the tip of your nose and then push that thought away quickly whilst saying the word JUST GOooohhhhhhhhh in your mind and seeing that thought being expelled and disappear as it spreads out vanishing from the area of focus that is our mind.

You can now try this now just sitting with your eyes OPEN and then go on to try this just walking. Then if you're at work or in a situation where it is harder to control your environment you can also try this here whilst looking colleagues straight in the eye – no one will ever know! If you feel it's just not possible in a busy work environment you can take yourself off to a toilet and spend a few minutes on your own practicing mindfulness to help you deal with anxiety anywhere!

Mindfulness Exercise to Calm the Mind

The best way to learn this is to again practice a very simple exercise to perform as an adult, give this a try now and you'll see just how simple and effective the process is:

Difficulty: Easy

Time Required: 2-5 minutes

Do NOT lie down or sit down – first of all just stand still, DON'T think about how your standing or if your shoulders are relaxed and dropped etc.

Do NOT close your eyes – keep your eyes OPEN.

Do NOT focus your attention on your breathing. simply pay attention to any thoughts that come into your mind.

Now focus your attention onto the tip of your nose without looking at down at your nose, just look straight ahead or anywhere you chose.

Anytime you notice that a thought comes into your mind no matter what that thought is, focus the energy at the tip of your nose and say in your mind with your eyes open 'JUST GO'..... and imagine pushing that energy like a cone from the tip of your nose outward and pushing that thought out of your mind.

With a little practice you will see the thought just vanish. As you say JUST GO you can also breathe out calmly using your breathe to push the thought away too making an Ohhhhhhhhhhh sound.

As another thought enters your mind (which it will) just refocus your attention on the tip of your nose again and push that thought away with JUST GOooohhhhhhhhhh. All our minds wander it's completely normal, so don't worry when it does.

The more you practice JUST GOooohhhhhhhhhh pushing the thoughts away the longer the gap will be in between each new thought arriving, and as such we are learning to take back control and calm our mind simply and easily!

When you feel you've mastered this which won't take long – it's very simple, then go outside and now repeat the exercise whilst walking. Allow the thoughts to come into your mind and push the thoughts away with JUST GOooohhhhhhhhhh as you walk.

If you practice this daily just 10-15 mins a day for 5 days in a row will help calm your mind and you will notice the difference!

You can now build this into your daily life, into your daily routine, but if certain negative intrusive thoughts come into your mind unplanned at an inappropriate time then you can use this at any time to help calm your mind.

How to Teach 'MINDMAGIC' - Mindfulness for Children

Teaching a child to use Mindfulness or MINDMAGIC early on in life is highly recommended, which is why it's now taught in schools.

There is a very simple of way of teaching children, and as with EASY EMDR we just use the magical world of spells once again! For many generations in many cultures magic has been used in TV and film to show witches and wizards casting spells to push away people, items and other spells or dark magic. We don't even have to look far to find very famous child characters practising magic to repel dark ghosts and ghouls using wands or even their hands.

All we need to do to convert the adult version to a child friendly technique is simply change the word 'JUST GOoohhhhhhhh' into to a spell – that's it!

In child Mindfulness we use the magical spell of 'PROTECTO'.

This spell is made up of the words PROTECT and GO and the O on the end replaces the Ooohhhhhhh as the effective sound that continues to push the thoughts away – 'Ooohhhhhhh'. That's MINDMAGIC! While Adults say JUST GO children can use PROTECTO it sounds more fun and more like a spell so engages the child's mind in a playful way which is essential with children.

So we teach the child to sit down and close their eyes and when a thought comes in they focus their attention onto their nose. You can tap them lightly on the nose to help them become aware of where to focus their attention but always tell them you're going to do this before you do and remember always ask permission before you touch a child even on their nose!

As the child focuses their attention onto their nose this becomes their 'wand' and they can then from the tip of their wand (or nose) as a thought comes into their mind cast the spell 'PROTECTO' out loud and push the thought away. Once they've mastered this out loud they can then be directed to learn how to say this spell in the quiet of their mind. You can teach children to use this during the day, at school and even at night which I have found highly effective in helping families teach their children to sleep tight at night.

MIND MAGIC - An Exercise for Children

The best way to explain MIND MAGIC is for the adult to carry out this very simple exercise with the child at the same time. You can do this one on one or as a group, so the whole family can take part at the same time.

Give this a try now and you'll see just how simple and effective MIND MAGIC really is.

Difficulty: Easy

Time Required: 10 minutes

Find a comfortable space sitting down together.

Explain to the child what your about to do. You can use the magical explanation that "sometimes when dark magic or thoughts come into or mind they make us feel sad or scared and that's normal, but we have a very special spell to make the dark magic go away and that spell is PROTECTO".

Practice saying the spell 'PROTECTO' now, make sure the spell is said quietly and not shouted out which it may do at first. Get used to saying the spell 'PROTECTO' over and over.

Once the child has mastered this then try breathing out on the O making it longer as the breathe is pushed out in front making a 'Ooohhhhhhhhhh' sound.

Now practice casting the spell 'PROTECTOoohhhhhhhhhh' breathing out.

Now invite the child or everyone taking part to 'CLOSE THE EYES'.

Invite the child or everyone taking part to breathe in and out and in and out three times slowly as we have already learnt and practiced.

Invite the child or everyone taking part to now focus on their breathing and experience what it's feels like in the body to slowly breathe in and out.

Invite the child or everyone taking part to now focus their attention on the tip of the nose. Ask permission first then lightly touch the child's nose reminding them to focus on the tip of their nose 'JUST THERE'.

Now tell the child or everyone taking part when a thought comes into their mind no matter what that thought is to say the spell 'PROTECTO'.

Invite the child or everyone taking part to PUSH THE THOUGHT AWAY using the energy at the tip of the nose as they say quietly out loud 'PROTECTOoohhhhhhh' and imagine pushing that thought out of their mind with their mind energy and their breathe.

With a little practice they will see the thoughts just vanish again and again.

Remind everyone taking part if they forget about what they are doing just to focus on the tip of their nose again and wait for the next thought to come in and then use the spell 'PROTECTO' again and again.

Remember to explain to everyone that all our minds wander off when we do this and it's completely normal, so don't worry when it does, just refocus.

The more you practice 'PROTECTO' with family and children pushing the thoughts away, the longer the gap will be in between each new thought arriving, as such we are teaching children to take back control at an early age and calm their minds simply and easily!

Continue as long as you would all like but 10-15 mins is very beneficial – especially if you practice this daily! Just 10-15 mins a day for 5 days in a row will help calm a child's mind and you will ALL notice the difference!

You can then use this at night if children can't sleep to help them drift off. It's based on the same principle as 'counting sheep' and so there's nothing new about what we are doing here, all we have done is make the process 'magical' to help engage the child's mind in a playful way. As we recap on what Dr Francine Shapiro PHD the founder of EMDR we can now equally apply this to both EMDR and MINDFULNESS: "Children are highly susceptible to EMDR, the complexity comes with engaging the child's mind with suitable play to be able to understand and adhere to the process".

Chapter 19

Anxiety & Depression Tests

If you would like to take a simple test to determine the level of anxiety or depression you or anyone else may be suffering from then there are two Self-diagnostic tests which are available for free on line or you can take them here.

They are not clinical diagnostic tests used by doctors and psychiatrists to make a formal diagnosis, but they can be used as a basic benchmark test to see where you start from, and after treatment with EMDR and MINDFULNESS where you finish up.

This is often very helpful for people to gain recognition and corroboration that what they are actually feeling is real and that change has indeed be made. By using these simple tests before and after treatment people often find the positive approval they seek that it has worked!

These tests are the GAD-7 for Anxiety and PHQ-9 for Depression.

GAD-7 Test

Over the last 2 weeks, how often have you been bothered by the following?

Not at all (0) Several days (1) Over half the days (2) Almost daily (3)

1. Feeling nervous, anxious or on edge	0 1 2 3
2. Not being able to stop or control worrying	0 1 2 3
3. Worrying too much about different things	0 1 2 3
4. Trouble relaxing	0 1 2 3
5. Being so restless that it is hard to sit still	0 1 2 3
6. Becoming easily annoyed or irritable	0 1 2 3
7. Feeling afraid as if something awful might happen	0 1 2 3

Add up the numbers to arrive at your Total Score   ____

GAD-7 Results – What does the total score indicate?

The severity of Anxiety is calculated by assigning scores of 0, 1, 2, and 3, to the response categories of :

"Not at all"	0
"Several days"	1
"Over half the days"	2
"Almost daily"	3

The GAD-7 total score for the seven items ranges from **0 to 21**.

TOTAL scores are placed into bands of 0, 5, 10, and 15:

0 - 5   = represents little or no anxiety

6 - 10 = represents mild anxiety

11 - 15 = represents moderate anxiety

16 - 21 = represents severe anxiety

Though this test is designed primarily as a screening and severity measure for generalized anxiety disorder, the GAD-7 test can is also recommended as self-diagnostic or home use test for three other common anxiety disorders:

Panic disorder

Social anxiety disorder

Post-traumatic stress disorder

When testing an individual for any anxiety disorder, a recommended cut off point for EMDR treatment is a score of 11 or greater.

So if the score is 11 or greater then you should absolutely consider using EMDR as it is the recommended treatment at this level.

PHQ-9 Test for Depression

Over the last 2 weeks, how often have you been bothered by the following?

Not at all (0) Several days (1) Over half the days (2) Almost daily (3)

1. Little interest or pleasure in doing things   0 1 2 3

2. Feeling down, depressed, or hopeless   0 1 2 3

3. Trouble falling or staying asleep, or sleeping too much   0 1 2 3

4. Feeling tired or having little energy   0 1 2 3

5. Poor appetite or overeating   0 1 2 3

6. Feeling bad about yourself — or that you are a failure or have let yourself or your family down   0 1 2 3

7. Trouble concentrating on things, such as reading the newspaper or watching television   0 1 2 3

8. Moving or speaking so slowly that other people could have noticed? Or the opposite — being so fidgety or restless that you have been moving around a lot more than usual   0 1 2 3

9. Thoughts that you would be better off dead or of hurting yourself in some way   0 1 2 3

Add up the numbers to arrive at your Total Score   _____

If you checked off any problems, how difficult have these problems made it for you to do your work, take care of things at home, or get along with other people? These will help to check against your results to see any improvements week upon week.

(Use "✓" to indicate your answer)

Not difficult at all ☐

Somewhat difficult ☐

Very difficult ☐

Extremely difficult ☐

PHQ-9 Results – What does the total score indicate?

These results help to indicate the severity of any Depression if present. This is calculated by assigning scores of 0, 1, 2, and 3, to the response categories

The severity of Depression is calculated by assigning scores of 0, 1, 2, and 3, to the response categories of:

"not at all"	0
"several days"	1
"over half the days"	2
"nearly every day,"	3

The PHQ-9 total score for the seven items ranges from **0 to 27**.

TOTAL scores are placed into bands of 0, 5, 10, and 15 and 20:

0 - 5   = represents little or no depression

6 - 10 = represents mild depression

11 - 15 = represents moderate depression

16 - 21 = represents moderately severe depression

22 - 27 = represents severe depression

When testing an individual for any depression, a recommended cut off point to start EMDR treatment is a score of 16 or greater. The table below for the PHQ-9 Scores and Proposed Treatment Actions explains why:

PHQ-9 Score Depression Severity Proposed Treatment Actions

0 – 5 Depression Severity = None

Treatment Action: None

6 – 10 Depression Severity = Mild

Treatment Action: Watchful waiting - repeat PHQ-9 in 7 days' time

9 – 15 Depression Severity = Moderate

Treatment Action: Consider counselling, CBT & Watchful waiting - repeat PHQ-9 in 7 days' time

16 – 20 Depression Severity = Moderately Severe

Treatment Action: Immediate initiation of EMDR or other psychotherapy and consider immediate initiation of pharmacotherapy (anti-depressant medication)

21 – 27 Depression Severity = Severe

Treatment Action: Immediate initiation of EMDR or other psychotherapy and immediate initiation of pharmacotherapy (anti-depressant medication) seek specialist medical advice and, if severe impairment or poor response to EMDR, urgent referral to a mental health specialist for supervised management of the individual.

Therefore if you or the person you are helping scores 21 - 27 in the PHQ-9 test it is advised to seek urgent help from the approved mental health service for your area or country. Whilst EMDR can still be the main therapy or form a part of the ongoing treatment, it is vital the safety of any individual who may be at risk is assessed.

CAUTION

If you or someone you know is in crisis or thinking of suicide, seek professional help quickly.

Do not rely solely on this book:

Call your Doctor - or

Call the Emergency Services for your country - or

Go the nearest Emergency Room – or if these services do not exist seek assistance from a responsible adult

Chapter 20

SEEKING FURTHER HELP & FAQ'S

Do I need a License to carry out EMDR?

If you wish to charge for EMDR then you should meet the criteria as set out for each country, certainly you would need to be insured for which you would require a professional qualification. In the US only members of the EMDRIA can practice as professional therapists, even though EMDR is very simple. As long as you are not charging for your services and you do not advertise or make any claim to be a professional YES you can freely practice EASY EMDT at Home.

How long do I have to wait before carrying out EMDR?

The guidelines recommend EMDR for unresolved trauma beyond 3 months, that said there is a growing base since of evidence since 2018 to support the use of EMDR as an Emergency (even same day) Early Intervention, remember you cannot do any harm with EMDR so use EMDR as soon as practically possible.

Is there any age restrictions for EMDR?

Children from aged 5 may be suitable to undergo EMDR dependent on mental age and ability of the child to process thoughts.

Can I use EMDR on Myself?

It is indeed possible to use these methods to FIND, FEEL and FOLLOW your OWN fingers to FORGET trauma. The difficulty comes with breaking state, as you will not be able to ask yourself any confusing questions – as you will know what you're going to ask! Once you are proficient with EASY EMDR you can choose to tap your own knees which is easier than focusing on your own fingers. Visit www.EASY EMDR.com (not .org) for a self-help application.

You can also move your own fingers and FOLLOW these instead. It is even possible to close your eyes and imagine following your own fingers while you think of a traumatic memory. This is very helpful in bed of a night time if you cannot sleep – I do this often!

My arm aches when I carry out EMDR – what can I do?

This is quite common don't worry, when your hand reaches far left simply raise the other hand with your fingers extended allow them to meet, drop the arm you've been using and change arms. When that one becomes tired do the same in reverse – keep swapping arms.

The eyes of the person I'm helping become tired?

This is very common, just refer to the additional methods of stimulating the senses which is tapping on the knees and ask the person your helping to relax and close their eyes – the EMDR works exactly the same – in some cases even quicker!

The person I'm helping is finding it hard to concentrate?

This is quite usual as the EMDR will make it harder for a subject to focus on the memory as it fades in importance. Keep reminding your subject to keep focusing on the memory, you can also ask them to describe what they are feeling when the number has come down by two or three points - ask then what's changed for the number to now be at an 8 or a 5 etc? Carry on with the memory until fully resolved.

The EMDR is working really well can we do more tomorrow?

It is always advisable to leave at least 48 hours between each EMDR session. Keep each session to a maximum of 2 hours for best effect.

This section will continue to grow as more questions are posed and answered. To see the up to date list of FAQ's or if you are seeking further help then please visit www.EASYEMDR.org the online portal for support and help, where you can find on line video tutorials and further guidance.

In addition there are a further 8 specific titles in the EASY EMDR for EVERYONE EVERYWHERE series. These titles are designed to help specific groups of the population and there is additional information in each book relevant to each group

:

The Complete EASY EMDR SERIES

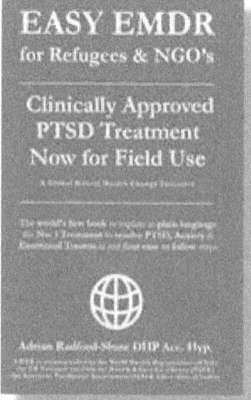

The complete EASY EMDR Series

1. EASY EMDR FOR CHILDREN & PARENTS

How to treat children aged 5-17 with magic and MINDMAGIC

2. EASY EMDR FOR ADULTS ONLY

How to treat adults includes MINDFULNESS for adults

3. EASY EMDR FOR WEIGHT LOSS

Treat the trigger causes of emotional eating and weight gain to overcome obesity and finally become able to get rid of fat and unhealthy foods – kick start your weight loss program effectively

4. EASY EMDR FOR ADDICTONS & OCD

Treat the trigger causes of anxiety to overcome addictions & OCD's

5. EASY EMDR FOR MILITARY & FAMILIES

For all service personnel, veterans and their families to resolve PTSD

6. EASY EMDR FOR ANXIOUS MOTHERS

A specific focus for Mothers struggling with anxiety and parenting

7. EASY EMDR FOR POLICE, FIRE & MEDICS

For Emergency Service personnel & their families to resolve PTSD

8. EASY EMDR FOR THERAPISTS AND CLINICS

A specific title for therapists to learn EASY Child & Adult EMDR

9. EASY EMDR FOR REFUGEES AND NGO'S

FREE for NGO's to treat child & adult War & Displacement trauma

ABOUT THE AUTHOR

Meet Adrian Radford-Shute DHP Acc. Hyp.

Adrian is a fully qualified and registered professional EMDR & Clinical Hypnotherapy Specialist Practitioner, with private clinics in London, Hitchin and Northampton, where he has since 2014 been practising EMDR privately full time, after he had witnessed first-hand his own full resolution of Complex PTSD by the treatment of EMDR, after every other psychotherapy and drug therapy failed, one of the reasons why he changed his career entirely to help treat others.

Through his extensive positive personal experiences with EMDR, Adrian has for the last 5 years helped children, adults and families regain control of their own lives from the exceptionally challenging psychological and physical conditions in their daily lives and in their past caused by anxiety & emotional trauma with the EMDR treatment.

Adrian was formerly employed in the Intelligence and Security industry. Adrian began his career in the Intelligence Corps of the British Army and went on to work as a civilian trainer with US Special Forces and UK Government Agencies before embarking on a career in Media and Business Development.

At primary school age Adrian was a victim of non-family child abuse which he then struggled to keep secret for over 35 years, unable to come to terms with the emotional and psychological trauma. Adrian suffered in silence with anxiety, an eating disorder, obesity, unhappiness and an overwhelming sense of a lack of self-worth. As a result in adulthood he strived to be a perfectionist to compensate for the hurt and anger experienced in his childhood.

He literally almost then worked himself to his death to succeed in a highly successful award winning career. Following the murder of his step Father and at the same time gaining the knowledge his abuser had died in a car accident, he finally confided in his family only to find out his abuser had not died – it was another acquaintance of the family. His abuser was still alive and everyone now knew! Distraught with uncontrollable emotion he finally sought help from the mental health services.

Adrian was referred to the NHS for counselling but received only one assessment interview. At that time it was explained to him frankly the mental health services in the UK had no real ability to help adult survivors of child abuse, and so it was suggested he fly out that week to a private American survivors clinic instead.

Adrian was however fully covered with a gold standard armed forces veterans private health insurance policy, and once again he was refused any help. Adrian made a formal complaint which lasted 8 weeks where upon the complaint was found in his favour, in that private insurance does cover mental health. Adrian considers himself to be one of the few lucky people able to access private healthcare. He then underwent extensive counselling and therapy privately in the UK at the Priory Hospital, Roehampton where he was diagnosed with Complex PTSD.

Whilst resident as an in-patient at the Priory Adrian felt unable to find and make sense of all the memories jumbled up in his head. One day he realised whilst practising mindfulness, he was able to find clarity and focus and so took to drawing circles to record the thoughts as they unjumbled in his mind, and by writing just one or two words in each of those circles he was able to quickly map out his mind very clearly on paper.

Then after a group therapy session one day, the subject being Subjective Units of Distress (SUD's), Adrian realised he could then grade the memories in the circles he had drawn and he noticed when he sat with the thoughts, he could feel the anxiety present in his body, which related to the SUD's he had previously recorded.

This helped Adrian to identify and prioritise the target subjects in his mind which he was then able to take to his psychiatrist sessions. Whilst Adrian was not able to resolve these traumas through psychotherapy and counselling, he gained a full understanding of how to quickly and non-verbally 'pull out' deep rooted traumas mindfully.

Other patients became very interested in this new therapy Adrian had inadvertently developed, and they too began to draw circles, grading them and taking these to their own psychiatrists. The senior consultants at the Priory were amazed at how simple this new therapy was in identifying 'locked in' trauma and found they were then able to help their patients more effectively with a fuller understanding of the traumas their clients had experienced that they were until now unable to verbally communicate. And thus Memory Mapping was born as a new powerful therapy to expedite the formulation of a treatment plan for anxiety and emotional and psychological trauma.

Adrian was not treated with EMDR at the Priory Hospital and so all the traumas he had identified through his memory mapping remained locked in and unresolved, whilst other patients were able to finally resolve their own traumas. After a few months of seeing no progress Adrian was advised to visit an external and acclaimed EMDR specialist Edward Sim in Uckfield.

He was at his lowest point, suffering from frank thoughts of suicide, having to even be talked down on the phone from driving into oncoming lorries on his way to visit Edward for the first time.

Adrian arrived safely and underwent a two hour session with Edward. He was astounded at the immediate, powerful and highly effective results of the EMDR treatment as he became simply no longer bothered by the emotion he once felt when recalling all his past traumas. One by one he was quickly and efficiently able to desensitise himself form the all the psychological problems associated with his severe anxiety and emotional trauma - in just one session!

That same day Adrian on the drive home, free of any thoughts of suicide, reverted back to being the person he used to be, strong, confident, happy and anxiety free. Adrian describes this as nothing short of a miracle.

After a number of weeks had passed he finally found the strength to report the abuse he suffered to police who then took his abuser to court. The trail for Adrian was highly traumatic being forced to relive the details of the abuse over and over again. Adrian revisited Edward Sim for a further two hour 'top up' session, and after only 1 hour feeling his PTSD was again completely resolved he spent, at his request, the remaining hour talking to Edward in depth about a career as a therapist.

Through his discussions with Edward over EMDR having resolved permanently the underlying diagnosis of Complex PTSD, in the period after Adrian began to experience what is termed Post Traumatic 'Growth' rather than 'stress'.

After facing and overcoming so much adversity and with much personal experience of trauma (when he was also faced with a severe permanent and disabling physical condition) and with much experience of a multitude of differing therapies and EMDR, Adrian realised he had the ability to help others and become an EMDR therapist himself to give back.

And so Adrian went on to formally study Clinical Hypnotherapy and then EMDR whilst also studying CBT, Schema, Stress, Anxiety, Anger Management, Relationships, Bereavement, Assertiveness, Mindfulness and Weight Management.

Adrian soon realised his earlier work in the development of Memory Mapping could be integrated seamlessly into the standard EMDR protocol. Adrian began carrying out research on the use of Memory Mapping with his clients in therapy. The results were astounding with 100% of subjects being able to recall 'locked in trauma' in minutes rather than hours. Soon Adrian realised by using Memory Mapping instead of conventional time line therapies he had expedited the treatment process by 80% when compared to the NICE guidelines.

This had the effect of reducing the number of sessions clients required and thus the overall treatment costs. Adrian was able to therefore open up access to EMDR to the everyday person by charging far less - up to 80% less, removing cost as a barrier to treatment access. EMDR became affordable to the masses not just the rich or privately insured.

In fact the non-verbal Memory Mapping appealed to an even much wider audience where 'manly men' now felt able to attend for EMDR treatment because they never had to talk about or discuss their own traumas – they could in confidence just write codewords in circles, which were used as the 'labels' of memories to facilitate the EMDR treatment. In addition Adrian found that children were also highly comfortable with drawing and writing memories of trauma easily in circles. The realisation that Memory Mapping had revolutionised EMDR for the masses now became very apparent.

Whilst watching the Harry Potter films Adrian realised JK Rowling had, in using Mind Extraction and Oblivation spells, wands to pull out memories, memory flasks and magical memory reading devices, inadvertently woven EMDR into the magical world of wizards. Adrian used this as inspiration to devise the very therapy Dr Francine Shapiro PhD. wrote about finding to engage the child's mind with suitable play. And MindMagic the Child EMDR therapy was born!

Adrian went on to provide pro bono EMDR services to Kids Aid, a Northampton based children's charity helping children and their families overcome trauma with MindMagic and EMDR.

Adrian being passionate about the future of EMDR as he could see it as a global treatment for psychological trauma and anxiety as a home based clinical therapy, and so he went about further devising a method using his military and civilian training credentials to simplify EMDR into the 4 Step Home Use process we now see here today.

By simplifying his language in therapy sessions so his clients from non-medical backgrounds could understand the EMDR process, Adrian was able to formulate through tested and evaluated study the 4 step EASY EMDR clinical approach. The process was so simple it was suitable to teach Adults for home use and as such the global mental health initiative that is EASY EMDR for Everyone Everywhere was born. Now EMDR could be learnt at home, now everyone could learn and practice EASY EMDR and so families could now finally resolve the mental health issues within their own families all around the globe without the need to access expensive therapy, if they could access it at all.

Adrian realised that even so, some families and those people in most developing countries may not be able to afford the purposefully low cover price of the EASY EMDR books, so he established the UK's first and only EMDR charity 'PTSD FREE' to enable disadvantaged families in the UK and around the globe, and child and adult refugees suffering from PTSD through war and displacement gain access to EMDR through working with partners to facilitate access to EMDR.

At least 10% of the cover price paid for every EASY EMDR book is set aside for the printing of books to go to these families.

EASY EMDR is just the beginning of this Global Mental Health Change Initiative and we thank you for your support in promoting and funding the help needed by children and adults across the globe.

Welcome to the EMDR CLUB!

To get involved in this Global Mental Health Change Initiative or for media enquiries or to kindly donate please contact us at:

www.EASYEMDR.org

www.ingramcontent.com/pod-product-compliance
Lightning Source LLC
Chambersburg PA
CBHW051305220526
45468CB00004B/1211